Fatty Liver

You Can Reverse It

By

Sandra Cabot MD

and

"Confessions of a Fat Man"

An autobiographical essay by
Thomas Eanelli MD

Radiation Oncologist

Do not go where the path may lead. Go instead where there is no path and leave a trail.

Ralph Waldo Emerson

www.liverdoctor.com

www.sandracabot.com

www.confessionsofafatman.com

The information and procedures contained in this book are based upon the research and the professional experiences of the authors.

The recommendations in this book are not intended as a substitute for consulting with your own physician. All persons with liver problems should remain under the care of their personal physician.

First published in the United States of America
2010 by S.C.B. Inc. International
P.O. Box 5070, Glendale AZ USA 85312
Telephone 1 623 334 3232 or 1 888 755 4837

Distributed in the UK & Europe by
Roundhouse Group, Maritime House,
Basin Road North, Hove BN41 1WR
T. 01273 704 962   F. 01273 704 963
W. www.roundhousegroup.co.uk
E. alan@roundhousegroup.co.uk

www.liverdoctor.com
www.sandracabot.com

ISBN 978-0-9673983-9-6

HEA048000 HEALTH & FITNESS / Diet & Nutrition / General

HEA039010 HEALTH & FITNESS / Diseases / Gastrointestinal

liver, liver function, fatty liver, cirrhosis, diet, hepatitis, nutrition

ABOUT THE AUTHORS

Dr. Sandra Cabot

Dr Sandra Cabot is the author of twenty one books on health including the famous Liver Cleansing Diet book which has sold over 2 million copies and is translated into 6 languages. She graduated with Honors in Medicine and Surgery in 1975 from Adelaide University, South Australia. During the 1980s Sandra spent considerable time working in the Department of Obstetrics and Gynaecology in a large missionary hospital in the Himalayan foothills of India.

Dr Cabot has lectured for the American Liver Foundation, The Primary Biliary Cirrhosis Society and The Hepatitis C Council of Australia where she was the protagonist in the great debate "Does the liver need a good cleanse?"

Dr Cabot is involved in raising funds for women's refuges in Australia and is an Angel Flight pilot for disadvantaged patients living in rural Australia.

Dr. Thomas Eanelli

Dr Thomas Eanelli is the medical director of Radiation Oncology at Orange Regional Medical Center in New York's beautiful Hudson Valley.

He is the founder and executive director of the cancer survivor advocacy group known as "Citizens Reunited to Overcome Cancer," and an Appalachian Trail section hiking club known as "Las Tortugas" and philanthropic physician alpinist group known as "Caduceus Climbing Club".

Best known for his pioneering work to break down the traditional "stiff white coat" barrier which exists and isolates patients from their doctors and medical caregivers. His passion to help others who suffer the same pain from addiction related disease and gratitude for Dr. Cabot's work inspired his part in this project.

Contents

INTRODUCTION

Is your liver a ticking time bomb?

Fatty liver can -

- Ruin your health
- Make you overweight
- Stop you from losing weight
- Make you diabetic
- Cause cirrhosis and liver failure

This book will provide you with a plan to reverse fatty liver, improve your liver function and restore your health.

Over the past 35 years of practising medicine I have seen patients heal themselves from so called "incurable" diseases and dozens of common and chronic health problems when they concentrated on improving their liver function. And unfortunately, I've also seen patients lose their lives because of liver failure. The truth is, in most cases serious illnesses don't happen overnight. Your body produces warning signs and symptoms of a potential or evolving health problem. The problem is most people don't know how to interpret or detect these signals early enough to do anything about them. The most important thing is that you do not wait until it is too late!

Unfortunately I cannot claim to be a guru, a saint or a miracle healer, but I can claim to have a lot of experience in healing various types of liver disease using nutritional medicine. I cannot promise to heal your liver problem but I can show you the way to try effectively to optimize your chances. Fortunately of all the organs in the body the liver is most able to repair and renew itself but you need to give it the right tools – I will repeat this saying several times and it's never too late to try.

I felt like I had found a life program which is a tangible fountain of youth!

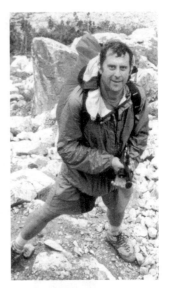

I have found the courage to tell the story of my food addiction - and how I found salvation and the tools I needed to help keep this dangerous addiction in hand - and it all started with Dr Cabot and her little green book . . .

Dr Eanelli after The Liver Cleansing Diet - feeling on top of the world!

For Dr Eanelli's full story see Chapter 15 - Confessions of a Fat Man on page 155.

CHAPTER ONE

Symptoms and signs of a fatty liver

Many people with a fatty liver are unaware that they have a liver problem, as its symptoms can be vague and non-specific, especially in the early stages.

Most people with a fatty liver will not feel well and will find they become increasingly fatigued and overweight, often for no apparent reason. Because the onset of symptoms is very gradual you may become accustomed to feeling generally unwell and slowing down. The state of your liver has a big impact on your state of mind so that those with fatty liver may find themselves irritable and moody with a poor memory and difficulty keeping up with life's demands. Indeed depression and poor sleep may be associated with a fatty liver and these things resolve when we improve the liver function.

Many overweight people with a fatty liver suffer with disordered sleep associated with sleep apnea and/or severe snoring. Sleep apnea is a condition where a person stops breathing for a span of approximately 10 to 20 seconds while asleep. This pattern continues several times throughout the night, usually without the person even knowing it.

Sleep apnea causes a drop in blood oxygen levels during sleep which results in the following –

• Fatigue in the mornings

• Falling asleep during the day

• Low testosterone levels and thus a low libido in men

• Increased weight gain

• An increase in blood pressure

- A higher risk of heart attacks and strokes

Some of the great benefits of reducing fatty liver include a reduction in these sleep disorders and an increase in testosterone levels in men.

The symptoms of fatty liver may consist of –

- Fatigue
- Abdominal bloating and congestion
- There may be discomfort or pain, over the liver, which is situated in the right upper abdominal area
- Accumulation of abdominal fat with a "pot belly" and a roll of fat around the upper abdomen known as the "liver roll"
- Indigestion and intolerance of fatty foods
- Reflux and heartburn
- Hemorrhoids
- Fatty yellowish lumps in the skin and often around the eyes– these are called xanthelasma
- Overheating of the body
- Excessive sweating
- Body odor
- Bad breath and coated tongue
- Red itchy and/or dry eyes
- Itchy skin
- Skin rashes such as dermatitis, psoriasis and brown liver spots
- Acne rosacea
- Dupytren's contracture in the hands
- Redness of the palms of the hands
- Hot and/or burning soles of the feet
- Headaches, especially associated with nausea
- Gall bladder problems
- Unexplained weight gain
- Inability to lose weight even whilst dieting

- High blood pressure
- High blood levels of cholesterol and triglycerides
- Depression and unpleasant moods
- Sleep disorders such as snoring and sleep apnea
- Low testosterone levels in men
- Low libido

These miserable and chronic symptoms are your liver's cry for help!

Let's look at some of these symptoms in more detail

Abdominal obesity

Your excess weight is largely found in the abdominal area so that you may have a "pot belly" and a roll of fat around the upper abdomen. I call this the "liver roll". You may also have excess fat around your neck and trunk so that you have an "apple shape". This is known as "upper level body obesity".

Many people find that they put on weight once they hit the 40-year milestone. It can be infuriating, frustrating and perplexing – and it does not help when the doctor says "well it's to be expected at your age!" In spite of the same exercise routine and diet, you find yourself with the "middle aged spread". Various euphemistic explanations are often given – ranging from menopause, middle-aged spread, stress, too much alcohol, slowing down, poor metabolism, but so what? You still don't know how to beat it!

Well have you ever thought there may be a scientific and treatable reason for your unsightly "pot belly"? Have you ever thought that you may have a fatty liver?

You probably haven't but you should, because it's highly likely - indeed, it's the new epidemic affecting millions of people, and for many it's the reason why conventional low fat - low calorie diets don't work for weight loss.

Syndrome X

Many patients with fatty liver have a chemical imbalance in their body known as Syndrome X.

Syndrome X is a metabolic disorder associated with abnormally high blood levels of the hormone insulin. The hormone insulin is produced by the pancreas gland. The action of insulin is to put blood sugar (glucose) into the muscle, liver and fat cells.

In those with Syndrome X the insulin does not work effectively because the body's cells are resistant to the insulin. To compensate for this the pancreas produces more and more insulin so that abnormally high levels of insulin result. Insulin levels can be measured with a blood test – see website www.liverdoctor.com/flb and click 'Liver tests".

High levels of insulin promote weight gain for 3 reasons

- Insulin is a fat-storing hormone
- Insulin suppresses the production of fat-burning hormones in your body
- Insulin increases the appetite especially for sweets or carbohydrates; insulin makes you hungry even when you don't need to eat

High insulin levels are often associated with unstable or high blood sugar levels. Indeed you may be pre-diabetic. Those with Syndrome X often have abnormalities in blood fat levels (high cholesterol and triglycerides) and may have elevated levels of uric acid.

Skin problems

If your liver is not doing its job of breaking down toxins efficiently they must be eliminated from your body by other means – in many cases they come out through your skin!

These toxins can manifest as:

- Dermatitis
- Eczema
- Brown liver spots which make you look older
- Red itchy rashes anywhere on your body
- Hives
- Psoriasis
- Acne rosacea on the face – this typically affects the cheeks, chin and area around the nose

If toxins are excreted through your skin they will irritate and inflame the skin - rashes, acne rosacea, psoriasis or brown spots may start to occur. I have often found that worsening skin problems are a sign of liver dysfunction or of future liver problems on the horizon.

If the skin is treated with strong steriod creams to suppress the rash, the toxins cannot escape from your body and may cause health problems on a deeper level. Thus steroid creams must only be used intermittently for short periods of time. Commonly, acne rosacea is treated with antibiotics which do not work very well and, if used long term, will make your liver unhealthy and possibly damage your liver. Acne rosacea can be treated with tea tree oil body wash instead of soap and this will control infection. A good liver tonic (see page 41), omega 3 supplements and raw juices are essential to make your skin healthy again.

High blood pressure

Poor liver function can trigger high blood pressure in several ways and I have seen many patients come off blood pressure medications and diuretics when they improve their liver function and lose weight. Of course I have to mention exercise, as it is a great way of lowering high blood pressure as well. If the liver is fatty, chances are that you have abnormally high blood levels of the bad LDL cholesterol and triglyceride fats. These fats make your blood thick and sticky and thus the blood pressure goes up.

The liver also breaks down the adrenal hormone called aldosterone, which regulates the balance of sodium and potassium in your body. Excessive aldosterone causes your body to retain sodium and lose potassium, which raises your blood pressure.

What's more, your liver controls the level of blood fats. Too much cholesterol and triglyceride fat can make your blood sticky and harder to pump through your arteries. This can also cause your blood pressure to shoot through the roof!

Dupuytren's contracture

This is also known as Dupuytren's disease or palmar fibromatosis and is best described as a thickening and shortening of the tendons in the palm of the hand. These tendons flex the fingers so the long term result is a claw hand and the fingers cannot be fully extended (straightened).

The ring finger and little finger are the fingers most commonly affected and although the middle finger may be affected in advanced cases, the index finger and the thumb are nearly always spared.

Dupuytren's contracture can be a sign of underlying liver disease that may not have been diagnosed and it can also be inherited.

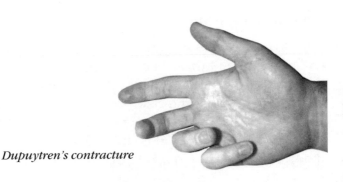

Dupuytren's contracture

CHAPTER TWO

Fatty liver – what does it mean?

During the 1990s I first recognized that the condition of fatty liver was becoming widespread as I began seeing more and more cases of fatty liver, especially in my overweight patients.

To me, this was a new phenomenon and when I trained as a medical student back in the early 1970s the condition of fatty liver was hardly mentioned. My observation of this newly emerging disease worried me greatly, as I could understand its serious consequences and yet surprisingly no one was talking about it, including the medical journals. Well it might be ok for geese to have fatty liver so that people can enjoy the delicacy of liver patè, but believe me it is not good news for you to have a fatty liver!

The liver is the most important organ in the body when it comes to your health and longevity.

Take the letter "r" off the end of the word liver and what does it say – it says live! If you wish to have a long and healthy life you need to have a healthy liver. A fatty liver is far from healthy, as basically it is being choked with unhealthy fat building up within it. The liver cells and the spaces that form the structure of the liver filter become swollen and distorted with unhealthy fat so that they cannot function efficiently.

The healthy liver is a highly organized mechanical filter, which cleanses the blood stream so that healthy clean blood returns to the heart. If the filter is blocked with unhealthy toxic fat, the blood cannot flow easily through its spaces, and thus it is not cleansed. Thus the blood returning to the heart becomes full of unhealthy fats and toxins, which can damage your heart and your immune system.

The healthy liver filter removes and destroys the following in your blood stream –

- Dead and unhealthy cells
- Cancer cells – thus reducing the chance of cancer spreading
- Toxic chemicals and heavy metals which are contaminating our food, water and air
- Micro-organisms such as bacteria, parasites and fungi
- Globules of fat (known as chylomicrons)

If these things are not removed because your liver is swollen with fat, your immune system will become overloaded and you will age more rapidly.

My first observations during the 1990s of the emerging new epidemic of fatty liver prompted me to research the liver in depth and write the now famous Liver Cleansing Diet Book which has helped hundreds of thousands of people. The Liver Cleansing Diet is an 8-week cleansing diet, which detoxifies the liver and bowels.

I have decided to write this book specifically on fatty liver because those who find themselves with this condition need more specific information on how to reverse a fatty liver. They need simple and easy guidelines to provide a road map for life to keep their liver healthy. This book provides easy menu plans, as well as foods and supplements that heal the liver and specific recipes to remove the deadly fat from their liver. There are plenty of salad and soup recipes including my famous liver healing and regenerative soup.

In the Medical Observer Journal in July 2004, I read an article titled "Non-alcoholic fatty liver disease is the new epidemic of liver disease facing the Western world". Well it has been gradually creeping upon us, but in reality it has

THE LIVER

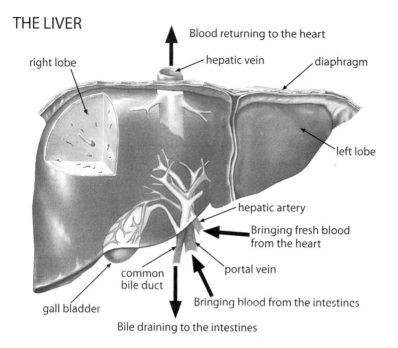

right lobe

Blood returning to the heart

hepatic vein

diaphragm

left lobe

hepatic artery

Bringing fresh blood from the heart

portal vein

common bile duct

gall bladder

Bringing blood from the intestines

Bile draining to the intestines

been an epidemic for at least a decade now! Back in the 1980s fatty liver was mainly seen in alcoholics and rarely in children.

Today fatty liver is now recognized as the most common cause of abnormal liver function tests in the USA, UK and Australia. Around 20% (or one in five persons in the general population) in the USA and Australia has fatty liver disease.

Fatty liver has been described for years, especially since we have used ultrasound scans, but it has previously been viewed as an uncommon cause of severe liver disease. This view is absolutely incorrect! The severe long term results of fatty liver disease are being seen increasingly in liver clinics all over the world.

Fatty liver is a very serious epidemic because it can affect children, it can lead to obesity and diabetes and it can lead to cirrhosis and liver failure. Fatty liver will probably reduce your life span by many years and will greatly reduce your quality of life.

The severe consequences of fatty liver disease are now recognized and these complications are increasingly seen in liver clinics. Fatty liver will become the most common cause of severe liver disease and the need for liver transplant.

Thankfully the condition of fatty liver responds very well to correct treatment and is reversible. The trick is to pick it up before it is too late!

A fatty liver contains an excessive amount of fat, and the normal healthy liver tissue is partly replaced with areas of unhealthy fats. The fat starts to invade the liver, gradually infiltrating the healthy liver areas, so that less and less healthy liver tissue remains. This invasion of the liver by fat shares similarities with the way in which cancer tissue infiltrates the liver. The fatty liver is often enlarged and swollen with this fat and has a yellow greasy appearance. The most common types of fat (lipids) to build up inside the liver cells are triglycerides.

Fatty liver is known in medical circles as "Non-Alcoholic Fatty Liver Disease" and this is often abbreviated to NAFLD. The term NAFLD includes the condition of "simple fatty liver" but also incorporates the more severe inflammatory condition known as "Non-Alcoholic Steato-Hepatitis" also known as NASH.

It is interesting to know that NASH causes the same damage to the liver as that seen in severe alcoholics and this has been proven with liver biopsy. The increased amounts of fat inside the liver cells cause inflammation and this is mediated by free radical oxidative stress on the liver cells. NASH is a much more severe form of fatty liver than "simple fatty liver", because in NASH there is much more liver inflammation, and this can easily progress to severe liver scarring known as cirrhosis.

In the past it was not uncommon for patients to present with cirrhosis of unknown cause and this is termed "cryptogenic cirrhosis' because the cause of the liver disease was unexplained or cryptic.

We now recognize that many cases of these so called mysterious liver diseases are caused by the aggressive form of fatty liver known as NASH. Unfortunately these cases of fatty liver were never picked up in time to be treated and this is why it's so important to have the function of your liver checked with a simple blood test every 12 months. After all, we are talking about the most important organ in your body!

How common is fatty liver?

Fatty liver is very common where high carbohydrate processed food is easily available. The food keeps getting faster and faster and we keep getting slower and slower!

There is an urgent need to collect and document more accurate data on the prevalence of fatty liver.

The true incidence of fatty liver in adults is unknown because no prospective studies have been done. It is estimated to affect 15 - 33% of adults. This is a huge number of people!

It can affect people of all ages, and is not rare in adolescents and children. The true prevalence of fatty liver in children is unknown. Population studies have estimated 2.6 - 9.6% of children have a fatty liver and this increases to 38 - 53% in obese children. Cases of fatty liver in children can progress to diabetes and/or cirrhosis; this is very sad because it is easily prevented. The menus and eating plans in this book are suitable for children who are overweight and/or diagnosed with fatty liver.

During the 1990s hepatitis C was the liver epidemic that held the limelight for doctors, epidemiologists, and researchers, and although hepatitis C continues to increase and wreak havoc, the limelight has been stolen from it by the much more common and potentially serious epidemic of fatty liver disease.

CHAPTER THREE

- -

What causes fatty liver?

The causes of fatty liver include –

1. Incorrect diet is the most common cause, such as -

- Diets high in refined carbohydrates
- Diets high in unhealthy fats –see pages 30 and 31
- Diets low in fresh plant food such as fruits and vegetables and legumes
- Diets low in antioxidant nutrients, especially the antioxidants vitamin C and selenium
- Diets low in good quality protein - see page 29

   It's interesting to know that the most common cause of fatty liver is too much sugar and carbohydrate and not dietary cholesterol. A high carbohydrate diet will cause your body to become resistant to the hormone insulin, which regulates the metabolism of carbohydrates and fat in your body. Thus the insulin levels rise and the high insulin levels tell your body, and especially your liver, to store more fat.

   Lack of exercise will make you insulin resistant if you have a high carbohydrate diet. Insulin resistance and high insulin levels are known as Syndrome X. Syndrome X is also known as the metabolic syndrome and is the most common cause of fatty liver disease today.

2. Liver damage from prescribed medications such as some anti-inflammatory drugs, immuno-suppressants, analgesics, and cholesterol lowering drugs etc. Drugs that may contribute to fatty liver include – Amiodarone,

Perhexiline, acetaminophen (paracetamol), some calcium channel blockers, methotrexate, chloroquine, hycanthone, synthetic oestrogens, the glitazone drugs used in diabetes and Tamoxifen. This list is not exhaustive and some people can have very severe unusual reactions to drugs that other people do not have; these are called idiosyncratic drug reactions. Always check with your doctor if you are taking long term medications, to find out if they have potential side effects on your liver. If they do, make sure that you have a regular liver function test, and if any damage shows up, your doctor can change your medications to more liver-friendly types of drugs.

3. Liver damage from recreational drugs such as alcohol, narcotics, and amphetamines etc, especially as huge doses of these substances may be used in addicted persons.

4. Liver damage from exposure to environmental toxins such as solvents, dyes, plastics, glues, insecticides, pesticides, dry cleaning fluids, harsh detergents and many industrial chemicals.

   I am amazed at just how little care some people take of their liver; they do not wear gloves or masks when handling poisons and they use insecticides to great excess. I often watch in horror as some of the people I work with, heat their food in a plastic container, covered with plastic wrap in a microwave oven. Well the over use of microwave ovens in itself has unknown dangers, but if you heat food in plastic containers in a microwave, your liver may be exposed to plastic.

5. Family history of diabetes, fatty liver or cryptogenic cirrhosis increases your risk of developing a fatty liver.

6. Being overweight and/or diabetic increases your risk of fatty liver, and fatty liver is present in 57-74% of obese individuals. Fatty liver is found in 95% of

patients undergoing surgery for morbid obesity. This association can be compared to the "chicken and the egg" relationship. In other words, what comes first? In the majority of cases the fatty liver leads to being overweight in the first place and then the excess weight makes the fatty liver progress to a more severe degree. This is why it's so hard for overweight persons with a fatty liver to lose weight, unless they first improve their liver function.

7. Gastric bypass surgery (jejuno-ileal bypass) for the treatment of morbid obesity can cause fatty liver.

Thus you can see that there are several possible causes of fatty liver disease, and in some sufferers there are multiple causes acting together.

It is thought that those with the more benign condition of "simple fatty liver", will only progress to the more severe form of fatty liver known as NASH, if they experience other insults to their liver. This could include the use of liver toxic drugs, poor diabetic control, infections, excess iron in the body, lack of oxygen, heavy smoking or exposure to toxic chemicals.

CHAPTER FOUR

How do we first discover a fatty liver?

Your liver is the most important organ in your body.

The liver is the largest internal organ, located on the right upper side of your abdomen and is protected by your lower ribs. It weighs approximately 4 pounds (1.8 kg) in an adult and it can be a lot more if it's swollen with fat!

The liver performs hundreds of functions and chemical reactions every hour to keep you healthy and alive:

- Manufactures a quart of bile everyday to break down fat in the intestines. You can compare bile to a detergent that gets rid of grease from your dishes!

- Filters nearly 100 gallons of blood every day to remove toxins, unhealthy cells, cancer cells and much more

- Cleanses and detoxifies pollutants and drugs. If your liver didn't continually remove metabolic waste and toxins from your blood, you would be dead in a matter of hours!

- Produces more than 13,000 vital chemicals, proteins and hormones and manages thousands of enzymes to maintain an efficient metabolism – no wonder the liver is important in controlling your weight!

- Regulates blood sugar levels to prevent roller coaster lows which leave you exhausted

- Controls the metabolism of fats and sugar along with the help of the hormone insulin

- Stores essential vitamins — including vitamins D, A, K and B12

- Protects your immune system from overload – indeed the liver in itself is part of the immune system

The Chinese call the liver "The General of the Army of the Body" and if your body was a corporation, your liver would be the president!

Diagnosis of Fatty Liver

1. Liver Function Tests

The liver enzymes are often raised and this is usually discovered during a routine blood test for a check up. The liver enzymes known as ALT and AST are commonly raised above normal levels, and this signifies inflammation and damage to the liver cells caused by the fat building up inside them. Typically the ALT levels are raised more than the AST levels.

For an explanation of liver function tests and their values see page 153 and website www.liverdoctor.com/flb and click "Liver tests".

2. Ultrasound Scan of the abdomen

The ultrasound scan reveals the shape, size and texture of the liver. The fatty liver has an abnormal texture which will be seen on the ultrasound scan.

The liver may be enlarged – the enlargement is often only slight and is due to the fact that the liver cells are being swollen with fat building up inside them. The medical term for enlargement of the liver is hepatomegaly; "hepato" meaning liver and "megaly" meaning enlarged.

An ultrasound scan of the abdomen is a test of great value, as it is good at checking the texture of the liver and will show the streaks of fat and sometimes fatty cysts building up in the liver. It will also show the presence of liver diseases such as liver cancer, cysts and tumors. For more information on techniques to visualize your liver see website www.liverdoctor.com/flb and click "Liver tests - imaging"

3. **Liver biopsy**

Liver biopsy is an accurate way to diagnose the severity of fatty liver, but a liver biopsy is not without risk and is not usually necessary.

See website www.liverdoctor.com/flb and click "Liver tests - Biopsy".

Important blood tests to have if you have been diagnosed with a fatty liver

Some doctors do not take an incidental finding of fatty liver in a patient very seriously, probably because it has become so common.

However, it is important to be thoroughly investigated with a range of tests, which you can read about on the website www.liverdoctor.com/flb and click "Liver tests".

You may also ask your local doctor for a referral to a liver specialist (known as a hepatologist) for a thorough assessment; after all we are talking about the largest and most important internal organ in your body!

The outlook for those with a fatty liver

If the fatty changes in the liver continue to increase, inflammation and scar tissue may build up in the liver and more severe symptoms will start to occur. The liver gradually becomes enlarged and distorted by the fat building up inside it and its ability to function is compromised. If nothing is done to improve the liver function the patient will become more overweight and their quality of life will gradually diminish.

There is a type of fatty liver known as Non-Alcoholic Steato-Hepatitis or NASH, which is a much more severe form of fatty liver than "simple fatty liver." In NASH there is much more liver inflammation, and this can easily progress to severe liver scarring and liver failure known as cirrhosis.

These outcomes could be totally changed around if patients knew how to use nutritional medicine correctly. Of all the organs in the body, the liver is most able to repair and regenerate itself and it is possible to totally reverse fatty liver disease; I have seen this many times.

With the program in this book you should find that your liver function is normal after 6 months. To totally reverse the cellular physical damage in the liver it may take several years, depending upon the degree of fatty liver that you have. However you will start to feel much better and totally rejuvenated within 8 to 12 weeks if you follow this program properly.

If you are overweight, the fact that you have a fatty liver, may make the weight loss slow initially; this is because it is necessary to remove some of the fat from the liver before you can start to lose weight efficiently.

A fatty liver has "forgotten how to burn fat";
it has become habituated to storing fat.

The removal of the excess unhealthy fat from the liver is a gradual process; this is why weight loss can be slow initially. However feel fortunate, as if you had not realized that you had a fatty liver, you would have become more overweight and probably diabetic.

CHAPTER FIVE

Treatment of fatty liver

Drug therapy for fatty liver

Conventional medicine is researching various drugs to improve the condition of fatty liver. These drugs consist of ursodeoxycholic acid (a type of bile salt) and the diabetic drugs metformin and the glitazone family of drugs.

Some of these drugs can reduce insulin resistance and may help patients who do NOT wish to change their eating patterns and lifestyle; however there are no drugs that have been shown to repair liver damage. Many of these drugs can have adverse effects upon the liver, so I do not think this is the preferred approach.

The liver responds so well to nutritional medicine and with a little motivation, inspiration and ongoing support, even the stubborn ones amongst us will find that it is not too hard to make the modest changes in our diet and lifestyle that are needed. It is important to take a pro-active approach and not allow the disease of fatty liver to progress.

Not all doctors realize just how serious the problem of fatty liver can become and the patient can be left wondering what to do.

If you have been diagnosed with a fatty liver it is vital that you follow a specific and effective program to reverse the fatty changes in your liver.

The liver is able to repair itself and grow new healthy liver cells and over one to two years you will be able to reverse the fatty damage to your liver and achieve a healthy normal liver.

If you are overweight you will lose significant amounts of weight within several months; however the liver will take longer to completely repair itself, but do not panic as by healing your liver you will add many years to your life.

Vital principles to reverse a fatty liver

1. Follow a low carbohydrate way of eating

A low carbohydrate diet excludes sugar, refined and/or bleached flour and foods containing these things. Avoid all foods with added sugar.

If you are overweight and find it very difficult to lose weight, it is more effective to exclude ALL grains for at least three months, or even longer, and be on a "no grain diet". You can replace these grains with legumes (beans, lentils and chickpeas), seeds and nuts. Grains to eliminate are wheat, rye, barley, oats and rice.

Carbohydrates to avoid -

Table sugar, foods with added sugar or maltodextrin, polydextrose, high fructose corn syrup, corn syrup, golden syrup, molasses, jams containing sugar, preserves made with sugar, candies, sugary desserts, chocolate (except dark chocolate), ice-cream, muffins, donuts, pizza, pretzels, chips, pastry, cakes and cookies. The best type of chocolate for those with a fatty liver is dark chocolate with a high percentage of cocoa.

Carbohydrates to minimize -

Flour, breads, processed packaged cereals, crackers, pasta and noodles, rice and other grains.

For natural healthy and tasty sugar replacements see page 39.

2. Increase the amount of raw plant food in the diet

Raw vegetables and fruits are the most powerful liver healing foods. These raw foods help to cleanse and repair the liver filter, so that it can trap and remove more fat and toxins from the blood stream. Eat an abundance of vegetables (cooked and raw salads).

Whilst trying to reverse a fatty liver and lose weight, restrict yourself to two pieces of fruit daily.

Eat a large salad everyday, or better still twice a day and use a nice dressing made with cold pressed oils and apple cider vinegar or lemon juice. Some people only eat salads during summer as this is the way they have been educated. Forget this habit, as your liver needs raw food everyday!

3. Eat first class protein with every meal or for a snack

Good sources of protein include –

*   Unflavored plain yoghurt (it does not have to be low-fat) and biodynamic or organic yoghurts are preferable

*   Eggs - free range or organic eggs are preferable

*   All seafood fresh or canned (avoid smoked or deep-fried seafood)

*   Cheeses – cottage, fetta, pecorino, ricotta, Romano, mature cheddar, parmesan are good choices

*   Poultry – free range or organic is best

*   Lean fresh red meat

*   Whey protein powder

*   A combination of legumes (beans, lentils, chickpeas) and raw nuts and seeds; you need to combine the legume with the seed and nut at the same meal or the same time, as this will provide first class protein which contains all

the essential amino acids. If you only eat beans or nuts by themselves, you are not getting the first class protein you need to control your hunger and blood sugar levels. This is why it is not uncommon for strict vegans to struggle with their weight and suffer with unstable blood sugar levels and sugar cravings. On the other hand vegetarians who include eggs, cheese and perhaps some seafood, find it easier to control their weight.

The benefits of protein include -

- It does not elevate insulin levels and therefore does not promote fat storing
- It satisfies hunger for a long time
- It reduces cravings for carbohydrates
- It can be used by the body for energy
- It builds muscle
- It improves brain chemistry to reduce mood changes and depression

4. Consume healthy fats

Many people with a weight problem or a fatty liver have the misconception that they need to follow a low fat diet. Indeed you need to consume the healthy fats to support healthy liver function and an efficient metabolism. The menu plans and recipes in this book are not low in fat but rather have been designed to contain a good balance of some saturated fats and essential fatty acids; the good news is this will mean you will not feel excessively hungry.

Your body and your liver need cholesterol to be healthy and if you don't eat any cholesterol-containing foods your liver will manufacture cholesterol to keep you alive. Your body needs cholesterol to manufacture vitamin D, bile salts, sex hormones, adrenal steroid hormones and to protect your brain. I am not a believer in very low cholesterol levels and those patients taking large doses of cholesterol lowering drugs often complain of side effects such as poor memory, muscle pain, stiffness or a reduction in energy levels and lower libido. Generally speaking if your liver is healthy it will make the good HDL cholesterol which controls the bad LDL cholesterol.

Unhealthy fats are damaged fats because their natural chemical and/or structural nature has been interfered with by man or the environment. Damaged fats are found in all deep fried foods, processed and preserved meats, lard, dripping, suet, partially hydrogenated vegetable oils and trans-fatty acids found in margarines and cheap cooking oils. Avoid hydrogenated oils found in processed foods and snacks (read the labels on foods to see if they contain hydrogenated vegetable oils).

Butter can be used in small quantities but do not overdose, as although butter is much better than all processed margarines, it is still very high in fat and easily becomes rancid. Avoid cream cheese and only consume small amounts of cream, as it is too rich for those with a fatty liver and often aggravates gallstones. Avoid cheap sliced processed cheeses as many contain added hydrogenated vegetable oil, colorings and additives.

You do **NOT** need to follow a low fat diet and indeed you need to eat the healthy fats found in seafood, cold pressed olive, nut and seed oils, eggs, raw nuts and seeds. Everyone requires omega 3 essential fatty acids for good health, which are found in oily fish, walnuts and flaxseeds (linseeds).

I myself take two tablespoons of purified citrus-flavored fish oil every day, as I am aware of the enormous benefits these omega 3 fatty acids exert on every part of my body, including my liver. Omega 3 fatty acids help to repair damaged cell membranes in the liver and reduce cholesterol and triglyceride levels. They also help to thin the blood, which greatly reduces your risk of the blood clots which cause strokes, heart attacks and sudden death. Although I do eat fish regularly, I find that I need the extra fish oil every day to feel really well and prevent headaches. The straight fish oil is more effective than the fish oil capsules, as it is easier to take the large doses required to reduce inflammation and thin the blood. It is important to keep the fish oil in the fridge and take it just before you eat.

5. Do not eat very large meals

If you have a fatty liver, eating very large meals will make you fatigued and bloated. After eating a very large meal you may suffer with reflux and heartburn.

6. Take a liver tonic everyday

Correctly formulated liver tonics promote the repair of damaged liver cells and facilitate the fat burning and detoxification functions of the liver; they can also speed up weight loss.

Researchers have discovered that silymarin—a powerful bioflavonoid antioxidant found in the herb milk thistle—can help your liver replace damaged or dead liver cells.

Studies conducted by the Center for Cancer Causation and Prevention at the AMC Cancer Research Center in Denver, CO also suggest that milk thistle provides protection from carcinogens that affect other organs.

– see Chapter 7 for more information on liver tonics.

7. Drink plenty of hydrating fluids

I know many people who are chronically dehydrated because they do not consume adequate amounts of the correct type of fluids. Hydrating fluids include water, herbal teas, weak black tea and vegetable juices. Conversely dehydrating fluids consist of alcohol, coffee, sweet or sugary drinks and diet drinks.

If you are well hydrated with the correct fluids, your circulation will be good and all your cells will function more efficiently. Your liver and kidney function will be optimized by hydrating fluids and your blood pressure will remain lower. Your body's acid-base balance will be better and will remain more alkaline, which improves detoxification and reduces the risk of cancer cells growing in your body.

Remember the liver is the filter and cleanser of your blood stream and the protector of your immune system. If you make it a regular habit to remain well hydrated your liver filter will be a much more effective internal cleanser. Staying well hydrated is also another method to increase your metabolism and facilitate weight loss.

8. A regular exercise program is important

Regular exercise speeds up the metabolism and reduces insulin levels. Why not join a gym or buy yourself an exercise machine that allows you to do weight resistance exercises? Walking, swimming and recreational sports can be incorporated into your lifestyle.

If you are very overweight and unfit, the best exercises to start with are gentle walking and swimming as this will not damage your joints.

Please take the time to do these things with the understanding that your health is more important than meeting deadlines at work or at home.

I have created a small gym in my garage where I have a treadmill, exercise bike and cross trainer to do upper level body weights. I find it relaxing as I watch television or listen to interesting radio shows while I exercise. We all need this "me time" that allows us to get into sync with our body.

Once you improve your liver function you will find that you have a lot more physical energy and that your mental state and moods are much better. Thus you will have extra energy to exercise and to achieve the things that you previously struggled to get through.

CHAPTER SIX

Appetite and satisfaction

For those people who think they may be addicted to food it is important to know that the most addictive foods are those high in carbohydrates especially refined sugar. Some people will also find that foods containing grains are addictive for them. Addictive foods can be called "trigger foods" in that they trigger an overeating binge and a loss of control.

Trigger foods set off powerful chemical changes in the body such as:

- High insulin levels
- Unstable blood sugar levels
- Low dopamine levels in the brain

These chemical changes increase hunger and reduce feelings of satisfaction; thus you need to eat much larger amounts of these high carbohydrate foods to feel satisfied and happy. In some people these high carbohydrate trigger foods, cause them to eat huge amounts, until they get to the point where they are unable to fit anymore food into their stomach, but still the chemical imbalances and the chemical hunger remain. This is why it might be imperative for such carbohydrate addicted people to avoid refined sugars and all grains.

Conversely foods that contain mainly protein do not set off these addictive chemical changes in the body and people do not tend to overeat protein foods. Your liver can turn protein into energy so that you will not get tired if you avoid sugar and grains. Protein foods contain the important amino acids tryptophan and tyrosine, which the brain uses to make its happy chemicals (neurotransmitters). The brain chemical serotonin is made from the amino acid tryptophan and the brain chemical dopamine is made from the amino acid tyrosine. Dopamine is particularly important for our state of mind, as it is the brain chemical that makes us feel satisfied, rewarded and motivated.

Some food addicted people find that using a tyrosine supplement helps them to boost their brain's dopamine level, which switches off their excessive hunger and cravings. Tyrosine supplements can also exert a worthwhile anti-depressant effect. Tyrosine can be taken as a powder or tablets and can be taken with water, juice or cup of tea or coffee. It should not be taken at the same time as protein foods, as this will reduce absorption of tyrosine into the brain.

The best friend of those trying to lose weight is protein.

Some weight loss diets are extremely low in carbohydrates and mainly consist of animal protein and green vegetables. Although these extremely low carbohydrate diets are very effective for weight loss, they are not sustainable in the long term. This is because they lead to constipation and increased acidity in the body and because they are so restrictive, people who stay on them for months may get deficiencies of certain vitamins and minerals found in a wider selection of foods.

It is extremely hard to live on a long term diet of animal protein and green vegetables, as you miss out of lots of delicious foods and will start to feel deprived and stressed.

The eating plan in this book is not extreme in any way and is designed to stimulate the removal of excess fat from the liver and to heal damaged liver cells. It contains a controlled amount of healthy carbohydrates mainly from vegetables, fruits, nuts and legumes. There are not many grain based foods included in these menus because we are trying to avoid high insulin levels and food addictive chemical changes.

If you have a very fatty liver it is best to avoid all grains and sugar for 12 months. In those with a moderately fatty liver it is best to avoid all grains and sugar for 6 months. Some people find it easier to decide to avoid all grains and sugar until they have lost all the weight they need to lose. Either way, you will not feel deprived by following the menu plans in this book because they include fruits, vegetables, nuts and legumes to supply the healthy non-addictive forms of carbohydrates.

For those who need more help with food addiction, also known as food codependency, see **Confessions of a Fat Man** on page 155 and the excellent book **Want to Lose Weight but Hooked on Food** *written by Wendy Perkins. Visit her website www.couragetochange.com.au*

Unstable blood sugar levels make you crave the wrong carbohydrates

Apart from alcohol excess, generally speaking, Syndrome X is the cause of fatty liver. Syndrome X is associated with high insulin levels, which cause the liver to store fat from dietary carbohydrate. Syndrome X leads to unstable blood sugar levels which fluctuate too much.

If your blood sugar levels fluctuate from too high to very low, you may need extra supplements to control them and this will reduce your cravings for high carbohydrate foods. When the level of sugar (glucose) in the blood drops to abnormally low levels, some very unpleasant and disabling symptoms may occur.

The symptoms of low blood sugar may include –
- Feeling dizzy and light-headed
- Sweating and a racing pulse

- Fatigue
- Foggy vision
- Moodiness
- Mental confusion
- Sleepiness
- Poor concentration
- Headaches
- Strong cravings for sugar and foods high in carbohydrates

The condition of abnormally low blood sugar levels is called hypoglycemia and this can be tested for with a blood test called a 2-hour Glucose Tolerance Test (GTT) – see website www.liverdoctor.com/flb and click "Liver tests - Glucose".

Hypoglycemia often alternates with high levels of sugar in the blood so that the levels of blood sugar resemble a roller coaster.

Natural supplements can be taken to improve the function of insulin and stabilize blood sugar levels; these reduce the symptoms of hypoglycemia.

The most effective ones are –
- The herbs Gymnema Sylvestre and Bitter Melon
- Chromium picolinate
- Lipoic acid
- Carnitine fumarate
- The minerals Magnesium, Manganese and Zinc
- The supplement **Glicemic Balance** contains all these ingredients in one capsule; it is best to take one or two capsules with every meal. For more information see www.liverdoctor.com/flb and click "Glicemic balance".

There are other herbs, supplements and foods that help with the control of blood sugar and these can be used in cooking or taken as supplements; they include –

- Cinnamon
- Nutmeg
- Fenugreek
- Coriander
- Turmeric
- Apple cider vinegar

Sugar replacements

If you crave sugar there are natural calorie-free and carbohydrate-free substitutes you can try – the better known ones are stevia and chicory root.

Stevia

Stevia is a naturally sweet herb, which has no effect on blood sugar and is calorie and carbohydrate free. Stevia is available in the form of powder, tablets and drops and can safely be used by diabetics. Stevia is excellent for those trying to lose weight but it has a very sweet taste and some brands have a slightly bitter after taste. Some folks love stevia whilst others don't like its taste at all.

Stevia is found in health food stores and many supermarkets. Synd X Slimming Protein Powder is sweetened with only stevia and is the lowest carbohydrate high protein whey powder available that tastes nice and is healthy. For more information on Synd X Protein Powder see www. liverdoctor.com/flb and click "Syndx Powder".

Chicory root

Chicory root contains a sweet fiber called inulin, which has been commercialized into a white powder called "justlikesugar." This sweet tasting powder can be used instead of sugar to sweeten beverages and to cook. Visit www.justlikesugar.com.au for recipes using "just like sugar" powder. Chicory root inulin does not contain carbohydrate or calories and is much better than sugar for those with a fatty liver or weight problem.

Sugar alcohols

Xylitol is a sugar alcohol which has 40% fewer calories and 75% fewer carbs than sugar; it tastes very much like sugar and leaves a cool taste on the tongue.

For more information visit www.xylitol.com.au

Erythritol is a sugar alcohol which has 95% fewer calories than sugar and is very low in carbohydrates. It is around 75% as sweet as sugar and leaves a slight cooling sensation on the tongue. Erythritol is very healthy for those with excess weight and/or diabetes as it has no effect on blood sugar levels and no effect on insulin levels.

Those who are addicted to artificial sweeteners especially aspartame and aesculfame, will find that by using these natural alternatives to sugar they can reduce their addiction. These artificial sweeteners can be very dangerous in those who consume large amounts regularly, especially if they have an unhealthy diet and drink alcohol.

See www.dorway.com

CHAPTER SEVEN

Natural Therapies for the liver

Liver problems, including fatty liver, can be associated with and/or cause modern day diseases such as:

- Obesity
- Diabetes
- Cardiovascular disease
- Chronic fatigue
- Excessive inflammation
- Autoimmune diseases
- Digestive complaints

Integrative medicine is finally starting to realize that these diseases are able to be helped by improving liver function. This has lead to a burgeoning of natural therapies available that target the liver. This is a good thing, as more people find the long term use of strong drugs to suppress the symptoms of disease has many side effects and dangers.

For someone with a fatty liver it can be difficult to decide what type of liver tonic will be most effective. This is especially true as fatty liver is considered to be a liver disease, which may vary from mild to severe.

I personally do not think it is good to take liver tonics in the form of herbal tinctures containing alcohol, especially every day, and on a long-term basis, as their alcohol content is not good for the liver.

After extensive research I found that liver tonics that are in powder and/or vegetarian capsule form are well absorbed and excellent for those with weak digestion.

Many people today take antacid medications to relieve excess stomach acid and reflux. Unfortunately these antacid medications reduce your ability to break down, digest and absorb amino acids from protein foods. Thus it is important to take a liver tonic that is easily absorbed and promotes digestive health.

The Livatone range of powders and vegetarian capsules contain combinations of specific liver herbs with synergistic nutrients.

I wanted patients to be able to take everything they needed in one formula thus avoiding the expense and uncertainty of having to swallow multiple individual tablets.

This inspired me to develop the Livatone range of liver tonics, which had essential herbs and antioxidant nutrients in the correct amounts, all combined together in one capsule or powder.

The Livatone formulas became a registered trademark so patients could know that they were getting my original formula with proven and safe ingredients. Subsequently several liver tonics appeared on the market with similar names such as Liver Tone or Livertone etc., but they are very different formulas to the original Livatone formulas and they do not have my name on them.

For more information see www.liverdoctor.com or phone our friendly and professional naturopaths in Phoenix Arizona on 1 623 334 3232.

Livatone Plus

Livatone Plus is a powerful liver tonic that combines the herb St Mary's Thistle with -

- All the B-group vitamins; these are essential for healthy liver function and detoxification
- The most important liver amino acids glutamine, glycine, taurine and cysteine, which are needed for efficient liver detoxification and liver protection

- An effective dose of the important antioxidant vitamins namely vitamins C, E and natural beta-carotene
- The minerals selenium and zinc, which promote detoxification in the liver and reduce liver inflammation.

Livatone Plus is a powerful synergistic formula that has been designed to support the metabolic detoxification pathways within the liver. Specific nutrients and herbs can stimulate the repair and renewal of damaged liver cells. They also enhance the liver's ability to break down toxic chemicals via the Step One and Step Two detoxification processes.

Detoxification Pathways in the Liver

Toxins ▶	Step 1 ▶	Step 2 ▶	Waste Products
(fat soluble)	*Required Nutrients*	*Required Nutrients*	*(water soluble)*
metabolic end products	B Vitamins	Selenium	
micro-organisms	Folic Acid	Sulphur	**Eliminated from the body via:**
drugs	Glutathione	Amino Acids:	
alcohol	Antioxidants	- *Glutamine*	Gall Bladder
contaminants	*e.g. Milk Thistle*	- *Glycine*	Skin Kidneys
pollutants	Carotenoids	- *Taurine*	Bile
pesticides	Vitamin E	- *Cysteine*	
food additives	Vitamin C		Sweat Bowel Actions Urine

Ingredients in Livatone Plus

Glutamine

This amino acid is high in organic sulphur and is required for the Step Two liver detoxification pathway which breaks down and eliminates drugs and toxic chemicals.

N-Acetyl-Cysteine (NAC)

This amino acid is high in organic sulphur and is essential for the Step Two liver detoxification pathway. NAC is the precursor of glutathione and is used in medicine to prevent acute liver failure from acetaminophen (paracetamol) overdose. Aldehydes, which are toxic breakdown products of alcohol and rancid fats, are neutralized by NAC.

Taurine

This amino acid is essential for the production of bile. The liver uses taurine to eliminate toxins and drugs from the body through the bile.

Glycine

This amino acid is required for the synthesis of bile salts and is used by the liver to detoxify chemicals in the Step Two detoxification pathways.

Antioxidants

The most important liver antioxidants are vitamin E, vitamin C, carotenoids and selenium. Livatone Plus also contains green tea extract which has useful antioxidant properties.

Antioxidants prevent free radicals from oxidizing the cell membranes in the liver, which prevents cell damage. During the liver detoxification of toxins and drugs, large amounts of free radicals are generated in the liver; antioxidants are needed to prevent these from causing liver damage. Vitamin E has been proven to reduce scarring in the liver, which can lead to cirrhosis.

The antioxidant mineral called selenium has been shown in numerous studies to reduce cellular inflammation and reduce the risk of many types of cancer. Recent research has found that selenium promotes the death of cancer cells. Selenium is also able to reduce the replication of viruses in the body and is a must for those with chronic viral hepatitis. In those at risk for liver cancer, supplemental selenium is vital.

A fascinating fact of physiology that you should know is that glutathione cannot protect the liver efficiently if there is an inadequate amount of selenium in the liver. Glutathione can be compared to a "liver warrior" that fights to protect the liver cells from damage and selenium can be compared to the sword that the warrior needs – without a sword the warrior cannot fight!

B-group Vitamins

Livatone Plus contains all the B-group vitamins – namely vitamins B 1, B 2, B 3, B 5, B 6, activated B 12 and activated Folic Acid. The activated form of folic acid is called L-5-methyltetrahydrofolate (L-5-MTHF). LivaTone Plus also contains Biotin and Inositol. These vitamins are essential for the production of energy in the liver and many folks with liver problems feel excessively tired. The liver is the metabolic factory of the body and thus optimal function is vital for you to feel continually energised. B vitamins are essential for both Steps of the liver detoxification pathways. Many people who consume excess alcohol or suffer high stress are deficient in B vitamins; this increases their risk of liver damage.

Livatone Plus contains activated B12 (methylcobalamin) and activated folic acid which are vital for people who are poor at methylation.

Methylation is an essential biochemical process which helps all other chemical processes in the body. If your body is poor at methylation, you will suffer with imbalances in neurotransmitters, energy production and detoxification. Activated folic acid and activated B12 are essential in people who are slow methylators. Vitamin B 12 is required for the liver to perform methylation, which inactivates excess estrogens, which can otherwise build up and cause cancer. A healthy liver is essential for efficient methylation.

Interestingly many strict vegans are deficient in Vitamin B 12 and the amino acid taurine; this can result in liver dysfunction.

Broccoli powder

Broccoli is a cruciferous vegetable, which contains liver healing substances (such as indoles and thiols).

St Mary's Thistle (also known as Milk Thistle)

The clinically effective dose of the herb St Mary's Thistle (also known as Milk Thistle), is the dose that has been proven to reduce liver damage in many European clinical trials. The active component of St Mary's Thistle is called silymarin and 420mg of pure silymarin is required daily, to get good results during the first three months of taking a liver formula. Livatone Plus contains pure undiluted silymarin (milk thistle extract). Some people promote silymarin diluted with phospholipids (a type of fat); however, I prefer to use the higher doses of silymarin.

More personalized help can be obtained by calling our naturopaths on 1 623 334 3232 or by emailing myself and my team from www.liverdoctor.com

The silymarin in Milk Thistle protects the membranes of the liver cells with its powerful antioxidant properties and stimulates the production of new healthy liver cells to replace damaged liver cells.

Modern technology has enabled all these ingredients to be combined together in powder or capsules; this makes it much easier to take and much more affordable.

To get the effective dosage of all the Livatone Plus ingredients, you need to take either two capsules twice daily or one teaspoon of the powder twice daily.

The powder can be stirred into fresh juices or water and although the B vitamins give it a characteristic smell, it is not unpleasant to take.

Once your liver function has improved and stabilized, a maintenance dose of one teaspoon of the powder or two capsules daily should be enough and is suitable to take long term.

Livatone

Livatone is an excellent liver tonic which contains a mixture of the herbs dandelion, milk thistle and globe artichoke combined with taurine, psyllium, barley leaf, carrot, beet powder and alfalfa powder. **Livatone** is very high in beneficial fiber for the bowels.

Ingredients in Livatone

- **Taurine** For information on this amazing amino acid, see page 44.
- **Dandelion** (also known as Taraxacum Officinale) has been used for centuries to help those with liver and biliary complaints and has been proven to be both effective and very safe. This herb is able to stimulate the flow of bile because it contains bitter substances such as taraxacin. Dandelion has antioxidant effects on the liver as well as laxative and diuretic actions, which make it useful for liver and gall bladder inflammation.
- **Globe Artichoke** (also known as Cynara scolymus) has liver-protective and liver-restorative actions. Clinical studies have established its value in lowering blood cholesterol and nitrogen waste products of metabolism. Globe Artichoke is of use in cases of liver dysfunction, poor digestion and gallstones. It has been used for centuries to enhance healthy bile secretion. Bile acts like the liquid detergent you use to wash your dirty, greasy dishes. Without detergent, you can't break up the grease and the dishes remain dirty. Without bile your digestive system cannot break up fats that can wreak havoc on your intestines and arteries.
- **Milk Thistle** – see page 46.
- **Lecithin** (Phosphatidylcholine) helps the liver to metabolize fats and reduces high cholesterol levels. Lecithin is composed of choline, linoleic acid and inositol. A choline deficiency promotes liver damage, which can be corrected with lecithin supplements.

Choline is helpful for those with fatty liver and high cholesterol and helps to prevent a fatty liver. Lecithin helps to protect liver cells from hardening and has been proven to help remove excess cholesterol that can clog up your liver and arteries.

- **Psyllium** is an excellent source of soluble fiber and has been shown to lower cholesterol levels by 14-20% after only 8 weeks; psyllium is probably the best cholesterol lowering fiber available.
- **Carrot, Beets, Alfalfa, Barley leaf and Psyllium** comprise the powder base of **Livatone** and provide a boost of chlorophyll, antioxidants, carotenoids and fiber.

Livatone regular powder is an excellent laxative and bowel cleanser. Servings of **Livatone** are one teaspoon of the powder twice daily in fresh juices or water, or two capsules twice daily with food. Commence with half this amount for the first week, and then commence the full amount.

While taking the powder or capsules ensure that you increase your intake of pure water to 8 to 12 glasses daily. This water should be drunk gradually throughout the day.

Choosing a liver tonic

When you have a fatty liver it is vital to take a formula that contains an effective dosage of the active ingredients. The ingredients should be standardized and pure so you know that you are getting the correct dosage.

So when choosing your liver tonic formula, choose wisely and check the types and the amounts of the ingredients in the different formulations available - you may get a surprise! Some liver tonics contain herbs in only small amounts and do not have any antioxidant vitamins, minerals or amino acids at all.

It's also good to get professional advice when choosing a liver formula. For more information call our Health Advisory Service on 1 623 334 3232.

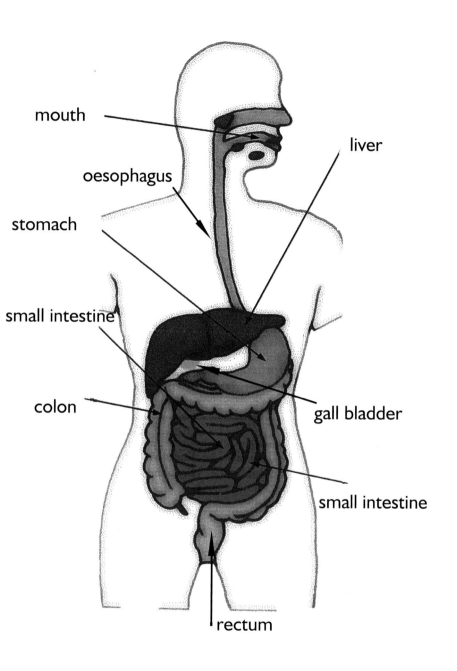

mouth

oesophagus

stomach

small intestine

colon

liver

gall bladder

small intestine

rectum

The liver is found on the right side of the upper abdomen - under the ribs and on top of the stomach

LIVER DETOXIFICATION PATHWAYS

Toxins ▶	**Step 1** ▶	**Step 2** ▶	**Waste Products**
(fat soluble)	*Required Nutrients*	*Required Nutrients*	*(water soluble)*

Step 1 — *Required Nutrients*
- B Vitamins
- Folic Acid
- Glutathione
- Antioxidants
- *e.g. Milk Thistle*
- Carotenoids
- Vitamin E
- Vitamin C

Step 2 — *Required Nutrients*
- Selenium
- Amino Acids:
  - *Glutamine*
  - *Glycine*
  - *Taurine*
  - *Cysteine*
- Sulphurated-phytochemicals
  - *e.g. found in garlic & cruciferous vegetables*

Waste Products *(water soluble)*

▼

Eliminated from the body via:

Skin · Gall Bladder · Kidneys · Bile

Sweat · Bowel Actions · Urine

Toxin List
metabolic end products, micro-organisms, drugs, alcohol, contaminants/pollutants, insecticides, pesticides, food additives.

HEALTHY LIVER

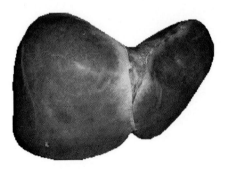

When the liver is functioning efficiently it is the major fat burning organ in your body. It is also able to pump excessive fat out of your body through the bile.

A healthy liver helps to keep your weight under control.

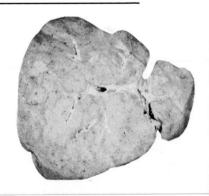

FATTY LIVER

A fatty liver is clogged with fat. It is unable to function efficiently and stores fat instead of burning fat.

It is also important to know that the liver tonic you decide to take is –

- Made in a laboratory that has obtained Good Manufacturing Procedures (GMP) certification and FDA approval
- Made in a laboratory that is audited by an independent not for profit body such as The National Science Foundation - see http://www.nsf.gov/
- Analyzed by an independent laboratory to validate the identity, purity and amounts of its contained ingredients
- Free of artificial binders and fillers
- Vegetarian so that the gelatin capsule cannot transmit bovine diseases

The **Livatone range** of liver tonics satisfies all these criteria.

Livatone Plus has been tested in a clinical study of patients with fatty liver and was found to be safe and effective. Ref page 245. More information on this study is available at www.liverdoctor.com/flb and click "Fatty liver study".

Since 1995, both **Livatone** formulas have been used in many countries and are manufactured in the USA and Australia.

Livatone Plus is a much stronger formula and contains far more ingredients than regular **Livatone** does. **Livatone Plus** is designed to support liver repair and promote the reduction of liver inflammation.

Livatone regular is designed to cleanse the liver and bowel and promote the healthy flow of bile.

Some people find they get even better results by taking both **Livatone Plus** and **Livatone** regular together - in such cases I recommend you take two capsules of **Livatone Plus** in the morning and two capsules of **Livatone** in the evening.

Livatone regular powder is an excellent laxative and bowel cleanser while **Livatone Plus** does not have a laxative effect.

Liver tonics are helpful if you -

- Are using prescription drugs – these must be broken down by the liver and many people are taking several drugs every day, which greatly increases the work load of the liver.
- Are using over the counter drugs, especially pain killers or paracetamol - these must be broken down by the liver and can be particularly liver toxic if excess or daily doses are used.
- Drink ten or more glasses of alcohol a week - over 18 million Americans abuse alcohol, making it one of the most common causes of liver disease in America.
- Smoke cigarettes.
- Consume sugar, fast foods, chemical food additives or a high fat diet.
- Live in a major city - where you are exposed to automobile exhausts, factory smog, crowded dirty places, water chlorination, fluoride and heavy metals etc.
- Use a microwave oven to reheat or cook your food.
- Suffer from a liver infection; millions of Americans suffer from liver infections — and many don't even know they are infected.
- Are over 45 years of age - as you get older the various tubes and ducts leading from and to your liver, as well as the internal liver filter itself, often become dirty and/or clogged. They become laden with unhealthy fats, toxins, gallstones, sludge, hardened tissues and waste products of metabolism.
- Drink soda pops and/or diet sodas containing artificial sweeteners, especially the sweetener aspartame – see www.dorway.com
- Are exposed to toxic chemicals and pollutants such as - insecticides, some antiperspirants, solvents, glues, aerosol sprays, some detergents, cosmetics, ammonia, hair dyes, nail varnish, disinfectants etc. – you may be exposed to these things at work or in the home.

- Do not drink enough pure water.
- Lack antioxidants in your diet.
- Have high cholesterol and/or triglycerides.
- Have skin problems.

There are many other reasons that would make it wise to take a liver tonic on a regular daily basis or at the very least, twice a year for a two month course each time. This is especially true in the 21st century when the world has become increasingly polluted and crowded, and liver infections are increasing.

Your liver processes most of the approximately 900 million pounds of toxic chemicals and drugs released into the environment every year. An overload of these toxins can easily wear out your liver and leave you prone to developing a range of health problems.

Be careful with pain killers especially acetaminophen (paracetamol), which can damage your liver. It is well known that overdosing on this popular painkiller can cause liver damage and death via liver necrosis and acute liver failure. A study, in the Journal of the American Medical Association, reported the highest recommended dose of Tylenol® (acetaminophen or paracetamol) can quickly increase liver enzymes in healthy adults. Elevated enzymes are the first sign of liver damage. If you drink alcohol or have kidney problems, the risk of liver damage from paracetamol is increased significantly.

Your liver is under attack 24 hours, 7 days a week, so it's vital to support its functions and reduce its risk of damage. If you have a clean and unclogged liver, you will have extra years of energetic living to enjoy.

CHAPTER EIGHT

. . . .

Testimonials for Liver Cleansing

Dear Dr Cabot,

I am in the seventh week of the Liver Cleansing Diet. As I told Christine, your naturopath, by phone the other day, the transformation of my mental and physical state has been nothing short of dramatic and life enhancing!

Your eating plan and Livatone Plus rescued a 47-year old father of two young children with diagnosed Fatty Liver Disease and has put me on the path to sustained heath. I thank God for your gifts as a healer - you have put an end once and for all to my unhealthy eating habits and given me the motivation to succeed. My wife says that I am beginning to look like the man she married ten years ago. Honestly, I feel better now than I did then, and I have yet to complete the diet! I have lost 10 pounds (4½kg) and several inches from my waist.

The most dramatic transformation is in my mental state; I am calmer, have more clarity of thought and am more relaxed. I just ordered your book Raw Juices Can Save Your Life and can't wait to try your recipes!

I was going to wait to contact you until after my cleanse, as you suggest, however, I just couldn't wait. You see I am a chef-owner of a heart-healthy home-meal delivery service so I love the idea of healthy food.

I like most of the recipes in your book, especially the brilliantly simple raw beet salad. I have been following the ingredients to the letter, however, I must confess that as a chef, I have been tweaking and adapting recipes to match my tastes. I made a grilled Ahi tuna over Buckwheat soba noodles with raw mung bean sprouts and shallots in ginger, garlic and wasabi dressing that was first rate. Your diet has re-acquainted me with the foods that I honestly love to eat but have been taking for granted. You showed me just how far off course I had drifted–too many midnight nachos and beer after a long day in the kitchen.

My company currently serves the entire USA under the brand Personal Chef To Go.

Yours ever grateful,

Chef Blair
www.personalcheftogo.com

Dear Dr Cabot,

I wanted to thank you for the good results I have obtained from following your program to reverse my fatty liver.

I began your program initially because I battled with excess weight for many years and had been diagnosed with a fatty liver. Well I was successful in losing 84 pounds (38kg) over the last 12 months and the ultrasound scan shows that I no longer have a fatty liver.

But the most surprising and unexpected thing to occur was the fantastic improvement in my skin – I no longer have psoriasis! This has helped my self esteem so much and I can now wear shorts and small tops and don't have to overheat under baggy clothes in the summer. I also found that the brown liver spots on my face and arms have nearly disappeared and that a scaly lump I had on my left cheek has gradually disappeared.

I did take your liver tonic, fish oil liquid and selenium as well and this might have helped my chronic skin problems. Thank you so much for making me feel attractive again.

Heather J
Pambula NSW

Dear Dr. Cabot,

I was 242 pounds (110kg) in August. I then decided to stop drinking beer and Chu-hi.

In September I received my Livatone capsules and the Liver Cleansing Diet book. On September 27th I started the diet and I kept to it. This Sunday the eight weeks will be up!

Well, after one week I started walking at night, then walking more with a little jogging; now I jog the whole 4k. I also started going to the gym 3 nights a week. Today I am 194 pounds (88kg)!

People I know are astonished. They can't believe it.

I want to get to 176 pounds (80kg). Next week I will have my blood checked. I am sure my gamma GTP, GOP and GTP will freak the doctor out.

I feel great!! But, one thing - Do you sell clothes on your web site? All my shirts and pants are TOO big! :-)

Thank you very much for helping me (and my liver) to get back to living life.

Nigel H

More feedback emailed from Nigel

Dear Dr. Cabot,

If I had not visited www.liverdoctor.com, I would still be sitting on the couch wishing I were healthier.

I was impressed by the testimony of Thomas Eanelli, M.D. What's so different about him and me? If he can do it, then so can I! So can ANYBODY with the right information. You gave us the right information - "The Liver Cleansing Diet."

The doctors I saw at the hospitals here gave me no advice. All they said was fatty liver.

I haven't had time to go back and freak them out yet, but when I do, I will have a copy of your book in my hands, and explain how WE did it.

I am not special, I have no super human powers - I just followed your advice. I know others can achieve what I did if they follow and stick to your advice.

I am at 187 pounds (85kg) now and this seems to be constant. I have heard of rebound weight gain, so I am continuing to eat meals according to your diet. I take Livatone Plus, MSM Plus Vitamin C powder and exercise every day.

Thank you, once again.

Nigel H

Dear Dr Cabot

I was not feeling too well and one of the symptoms was being extremely tired after working. I would fall asleep on the couch when I returned from work. My husband insisted that I visit my local GP and speak with him. He subsequently made an appointment for me to have some blood taken. A few days later he called me and told me it was urgent that I come around to his surgery and speak with him regarding my tests.

I was shocked when he told me I had Diabetes 2 and my blood sugar reading was 299, which is quite high. He wrote out a script for Diabex and also arranged for me to obtain a blood sugar reading machine together with needles and test strips. He also told me I had to lose weight and become involved in an exercise routine.

He then told me to phone the Fairfield Hospital and book into The Diabetes Educator Course which is held over three weeks. This all occurred about the final week in March 2009.

I visited the hospital on April 6 for my first meeting, April 20 second meeting and April 27 for the final meeting. Thirty people started the course – by the final session only around ten people were there including myself. I figured it all became too hard for them. At this final session, we were told we could lose our drivers license, suffer nerve damage, had a 50% greater chance of suffering a heart attack or stroke and could also go blind. I was shocked!

I decided I was not prepared to spend the remaining period of my life living like this. I am 63 years old and have up until then had excellent health. I did not take any sort of medication. My husband and I visited a health food store where I saw an advertisment for your book *"Diabetes Type 2 – you can reverse it naturally"*. I came home, made the phone call to order the book and eagerly awaited its arrival.

During this time, my blood sugar readings were all over the place from 180 right up to 346 – this was in the first week commencing April 7. I started to wonder if I would ever get well. These readings continued to fluctuate all through April, from 173 up to 301.

When I received the book I read it in one day and made an appointment to meet with your naturopath, Margaret Jasinska. My first appointment was at 10.00am on May 21. I was shocked after meeting with Margaret and told to change my eating plan to very low carbs, protein at every meal and lots of green vegetables and salad. Almost the exact opposite to what I was told from the Diabetes Educator. From that day I have religiously followed Margaret's instructions and have Synd-X Slimming Protein Powder with blueberries or strawberries or raspberries or kiwi fruit for breakfast. I take Glicemic Balance caps to balance sugar levels and reduce cravings.

I eat grilled steak, salmon, tuna and other fish at least three times a week, sometimes four. I also eat grilled chicken and duck breast with skin removed. I have roast lamb and beef. My husband grows all my vegetable and salad requirements for me, otherwise I buy them from the organic shop in Revesby. I also eat Brazil or walnuts if I'm hungry.

I had a second visit with Margaret, not sure of the date,

and she changed the number of tablets I take. I took her my blood results, which at that time I think were around 115. My doctor and Margaret were very happy with that. I told my doctor I intended to visit your clinic, as I was not prepared to put chemicals into my body over a long term period. He was very happy with this and said there is nothing wrong with alternative medicine.

At this time I have lost 53 pounds (24kg) and dropped several dress sizes, walk thirty minutes each day, and have not eaten one thing I shouldn't. I am still eating out at restaurants and just ask them to prepare my food by grilling it and not putting any sauces. I then tell them no sauces or dressing on my vegetables or salad – just a small serving of virgin olive oil on the side, so I can dress it myself. This is not a problem.

The most important news for me is that my doctor has told me I do not have to continue taking Diabex tablets and I just need to monitor my blood sugar. He is extremely pleased with my progress and said only a very small percentage of people attack the problem the way I have. Over the past month my readings have been from 74 up to 99. If I can continue the way I am going, I guess I can confidently say I have reversed my Diabetes naturally.

I am so happy that I went into the health shop and saw your advertisement. I refused to live the way the Diabetes Management would have instructed me to live and decided to look for an alternative healthy and natural way to approach my medical condition. I know I will always have to monitor the food that I eat, exercise and always make sure when I eat out I let the waiter know my requirements. However, this is a small price to pay for having back my healthy life and reducing the health issues associated with Diabetes.

Susie Sanderson

Sydney, Australia

Case history from Dr Cabot

Suzana came to my medical practice seeking help for recurrent discomfort over the area of the liver – meaning the right upper abdomen.

She brought along an ultrasound scan of her liver, which showed a lesion in her liver situated near the porta hepatis, which is the part of the liver where the blood vessels and bile ducts enter the liver. Thankfully this had a benign appearance and according to the radiologist's report looked like a type of liver tumor called a hemangioma, although it did have an atypical appearance. The radiologist had also reported that her ultrasound scan showed fatty changes in her liver consistent with fatty liver disease of mild to moderate degree.

The patient had been reassured by her local doctor that she did not have a cancerous or malignant tumor of her liver and that it was safe to leave it alone. Nevertheless Suzana continued to experience intermittent discomfort over her liver, as well as some indigestion and nausea.

Suzana had been on the oral contraceptive pill for 20 years and had recently ceased taking it, as she could not lose weight. I explained to Suzana that the long term use of oral hormones, such as the oral contraceptive pill, can cause hemangiomas in the liver. A hemangioma is a very vascular tumor made up of a group of enlarged blood vessels and does not become cancerous.

I started Suzana on a liver tonic and a selenium supplement and told her to drink a large glass of raw vegetable juice every day. She was to juice cabbage, red radish, orange, lemon, mint, parsley, basil, coriander, apple and carrot. I also put her on a low carbohydrate diet excluding grains and sugar and told her to eat plenty of raw salads and fruits, legumes, fish, organic eggs, nuts and seeds.

I gave Suzana a request form for a repeat ultrasound scan of her liver to be done in 6 months time and a follow up appointment during which I would review her liver function and symptoms.

Well, when Suzana returned 6 months later she told me a fascinating story and one that I had never heard before.

She said that one day she experienced quite bad pain over her liver area and had to go to the toilet to have a bowel action. When she looked in the toilet bowel before flushing away her bowel action she was shocked by what she saw. She described a yellow – brown gooey lump of material in the bottom of the toilet bowel that required several flushes of the toilet before it disappeared down the toilet drain. She said the mass in the bottom of the toilet bowel reminded her of molasses and she had never seen this before and said that it was distinct from her feces. After she had passed this gooey gelatinous mass from her bowels she felt much better and over the ensuing weeks she had no further pain over her liver area.

I reviewed her repeat ultrasound scan and lo and behold there was no sign of her liver hemangioma. Her liver scan looked perfectly normal.

My reaction was – wow! Congratulations you have given birth to a liver tumor! Perhaps I have a strange sense of humor but it really was quite amazing to see her completely normal liver scan.

As I always say, of all the organs in the body, the liver is most able to repair and regenerate itself.

CHAPTER NINE

Menu Plan to Combat Fatty Liver Syndrome

This is a carefully and scientifically planned way of eating, which is designed to –

- Reduce the amount of unhealthy fat in the liver
- Repair liver damage
- Improve the function of insulin and lower blood sugar levels
- Make weight loss easier and sustainable
- Reduce addictive eating habits

I have used it for over 30 years in my own medical practice and weight loss clinics with excellent long term results.

In my own practice I work with a team of naturopaths and we provide support and education to our patients. This education covers their diet, lifestyle, exercise and behavior patterns. We have a counselor who specializes in food addiction and addictive thinking patterns. Her name is Wendy Perkins and she has written an excellent book titled Want to Lose Weight – But Hooked on Food? For assistance, you can email Wendy at counsellor@scoastnet.com.au.

You can also visit Dr Eanelli's website www.confessionsofafatman.com for more information.

With your meals it is ideal to include –

1. **Raw plant food**, especially raw vegetables. A maximum of 2 pieces of fruit daily are allowed while you are trying to lose weight. After you have achieved your healthy and desired weight, you can increase the fruit intake up to a maximum of 4 pieces daily.

I have come across a lot of patients who suffer with a fatty dysfunctional liver, not because they overeat, but simply because they never eat any raw vegetables, fruits, nuts or seeds. Mostly everything they eat is processed and comes out of a packet. They get a shock to learn that a lack of raw unprocessed natural foods in itself can lead to liver disease. Sometimes I tell them to act like a rabbit - try eating plants and see the difference! I have even thought of getting dressed up in a Bugs Bunny outfit to motivate and surprise them!

2. **Cooked vegetables of different varieties** including some starchy vegetables such as carrots, parsnips, sweet potatoes, turnips and beets. This will compensate for the fact that you will not be eating much grain based food such as bread and pasta and you will need to avoid cookies and sugary desserts. Cooked vegetables may be excluded at breakfast or lunch if desired for convenience sake. Green vegetables contain much less carbohydrate than starchy vegetables, but starchy vegetables are still in an unprocessed natural form, which is much easier for the liver to metabolize.

3. **First class protein** because it will satisfy your hunger and does not lead to weight gain. Your body is able to utilize protein without needing insulin - that's why protein is slimming. For good choices of protein see page 29.

Extra Tips:

Satisfy your hunger

You may eat enough to satisfy your natural hunger at every meal and snack. Those who work in occupations requiring high physical exertion or those who do a lot of sport will need to eat larger amounts. Listen to your body and follow your natural instincts when it comes to the amount of food you need to eat to feel satisfied and happy. It is not how much you eat - it is what you are eating, that is so important for your liver and insulin levels. There are foods/ingredients included in our meal and raw juices recipes, which actually switch off hunger and lower blood sugar and insulin levels; they are slimming or fat-burning foods.

Quick easy snacks

Healthy in between meal snacks may include –

1. **Yoghurt** - plain acidophilus yoghurt is the best and it does not have to be the low fat variety. Make sure there is no sugar or artificial sweeteners added. You may eat ½ to 1 cup (approx 9oz or 250g) depending upon your hunger. The yoghurt can be eaten by itself or with one piece of fresh fruit (passion fruit is nice with yoghurt), or you can add 3 teaspoons of LSA or 2 tablespoons of Synd-X Slimming Protein Powder to sweeten it.

2. **Canned fish** in spring water or brine - sardines, salmon, crab meat, oysters, trout, mackerel or tuna – one small can (approx 3.4oz or 95g) mixed with the juice of ½ a fresh lemon or 1 tbsp of our healthy delicious mayonnaise – see mayonnaise recipe (page 103) and fresh chopped herbs. 2 Ryvita biscuits can be added but not if you are avoiding all grains or gluten.

3. **Cheese** – a lump (1.8 - 3.5oz or 50 - 100g) should satisfy you. Choose unprocessed cheeses as per our shopping list. The cheese can be accompanied with sticks of celery, bell pepper or carrot, or 10 olives, or 4 sun-dried tomatoes.

4. A **protein smoothie milk shake** (7 - 10oz or 200 - 300mls) for recipes see page 123.

5. One handful of **raw nuts and seeds** of any variety by themselves, or with 1 piece of fresh fruit or one piece of cheese (approx 1oz or 30g); fresh nuts are best and you can add salt to them if desired.

6. **Raw vegetable pieces** - good examples are carrot, cucumber, tomato, snow peas, bell peppers (capsicums), celery sticks or broccoli florets dipped into tahini, hummus or a dip (see dip recipes page 101 and 102). If you buy pre-made dips make sure they are free of sugar.

7. **Raw fruit** – one piece of fruit by itself or with ten raw nuts or one piece of cheese (1 - 1.8oz or 30 - 50g).

8. One bowl of the **Liver Healing Soup** – see page 90.

9. **Avocado Dip or Bean Dip** with sticks of raw vegetables or par-steamed vegetables such as broccoli, cauliflower or snow peas.

10. **One or two hard boiled eggs** – cold or hot with pepper and salt or curry powder or paprika sprinkled on them or mashed into them and ½ cup chopped fresh herbs (such as parsley and basil).

11. One small slice of one of our **Frittatas** – see page 127 for recipe.

12. A **raw vegetable juice** – one glass full – see recipes page 82.

Try to stay away from the following foods–

Sugar - Candies and chocolate which are high in sugar; some cheap chocolates contain hydrogenated vegetable oils which are most unhealthy. If you do indulge in a little chocolate the best types are the expensive dark chocolates and the guilt-free low carbohydrate variety made with sugar alcohols that are now available. Remember to use this as a special treat and do not overdose! Some people find it helpful to allow themselves a 'treat day' once a week.

Tip - You could have a square or two of a dark chocolate or a guilt free low carb chocolate with a coffee – it's better than adding sugar to your coffee!

Foods containing refined flour such as white bread, bread rolls, crumpets, muffins, bagels, cookies and donuts; they tend to be fattening and addictive for those with Syndrome X and/or a fatty liver.

"Diet foods" that claim to be slimming – they are usually low in fat and high in sugar or aspartame, e.g. diet yoghurts, diet jams, diet icecream, diet sodas, etc; these diet foods are not slimming; they are very fattening if they contain sugar or aspartame! Read the labels. For more information on aspartame dangers visit www.dorway.com

Fried and baked snacks – such as potato chips, tortilla chips, twisties, pretzels, etc.

Preserved meats and delicatessen meats such as salami, pastrami, cabanossi, fritz, etc.

Fatty take away foods like pizza, fried fish and chips, lasagna, fried chicken and all fries.

Biscuits and cookies – both sweet and savoury varieties, as they contain refined flour, hydrogenated vegetable oils, lard or shortening, and if sweet will be high in sugar.

CHAPTER TEN

Healthy Shopping and Grocery List for Liver Lovers

If possible try to buy produce that is –
- Fresh and/or in season
- Free of added sugar (read the ingredients on the label)
- Free of hydrogenated vegetable oils and/or trans-fatty acids
- Free of the artificial sweetener aspartame
- Free of chemical preservatives, colorings and flavorings

All of the above is not always possible, so do the best you can! Organic food that is free of insecticides is ideal but for some folks it's just too expensive and not always possible to find. So don't fret the small stuff!

- **Vegetables of all varieties**

  Vegetables that are highly liver cleansing are high in the mineral sulphur; these include cruciferous vegetables (broccoli, Brussels sprouts, cabbage and cauliflower) and bok choy, kale, garlic, chives, leeks, radishes, scallions, green onions and onions.

  Sulphur is needed by the liver detoxification pathways. Vegetables high in sulphur help the liver to break down fats and pump them out of the body via the bile.

  Fruits, vegetables and herbs with deep or bright pigments such as orange, yellow, red, purple and green colors are very liver cleansing (eg. carrots, pumpkin, citrus fruits, purple cabbage, parsley, coriander, beets, red, yellow and green bell peppers (capsicums), cherries, plums, mango etc. Their pigments are powerful healing antioxidants for the liver. Over a period of a week you should aim to eat a wide variety of differently colored fruits and vegetables so that you "eat the rainbow".

Alfalfa, barley leaf, wheat grass, kale and spinach and indeed any dark green colored vegetables can be eaten or juiced, or taken in powder form, to give your liver a boost of chlorophyll. Chlorophyll is the green pigment that gives plants their color and acts as a liver cleanser and source of magnesium.

Avocadoes, olives and eggplants (aubergines) provide healthy fatty acids for the liver, so include them regularly in your diet.

Starchy vegetables such as sweet potatoes, yams, beets, carrots, turnips, swede, pumpkin and parsnips can be eaten in moderation, as although they contain significant carbohydrate, they contain fiber and healing antioxidants, minerals and vitamins for the liver. Their nutrients are better absorbed if these starchy root vegetables are cooked. It is best to avoid white potatoes as they are too high in refined carbohydrate.

- **Raw fruits of all varieties**

  The best fruits for the liver are those that have a tart taste because they contain organic acids; these organic acids will lower blood levels of sugar and insulin and help you to burn fat. They also help to cleanse the liver. Fruits that have a tart taste include all types of citrus fruits, all types of berries (strawberries, blackberries, blueberries, raspberries, etc.), cherries, kiwi fruits, passionfruit, persimmons and stone fruits. If you are trying to lose weight, avoid or go very easy on the bananas, mangoes and grapes. Dried fruits are delicious and generally healthy; however they are much higher in carbohydrates, so if you are trying to lose weight, avoid the dried fruits.

- **Nuts of all varieties**

  Nuts must be fresh and good choices include almonds, macadamia, pine nuts, hazelnuts, pistachio, cashews, walnuts and Brazil nuts. Salted nuts are fine, unless you have very high blood pressure or heart and/or kidney failure. Roasted nuts are also able to be eaten in moderation, although not quite as healthy as fresh nuts, they are still low in carbohydrates.

- **Seeds**

  Seeds such as flaxseed (linseeds), sunflower, sesame, pumpkin seeds, chiu or chia seeds are excellent sources of healthy fats and protein. They can also be sprouted for salads.

- **Legumes**

  Legumes consist of beans of all varieties, lentils and chickpeas. These can be eaten cooked in soups, stir fries or salads or as a side dish. They can also be sprouted. Sprouts such as alfalfa, mung bean, wheat grass, barley grass etc are a good source of protein and chlorophyll.

- **Poultry**

  Choose from turkey, chicken, duck, etc - preferably free range and organic; make sure it is very fresh, as food poisoning from chicken is very common.

- **Eggs**

  Eggs are extremely healthy for the liver and have virtually no effect on your weight, as they are very low in carbohydrates and very high in sulphur and protein. Eggs have no adverse effect on cholesterol levels. Choose free range and organic eggs.

Eat plenty of eggs and watch your weight come off!

- **Seafood**

  Good choices include oily fish (tuna, trout, salmon, sardines and mackerel) and fresh fish (whole or fillets) and shellfish from unpolluted waters. Canned seafood is healthy. Avoid eating seafood raw, smoked or deep-fried.

- **Spreads for breads/crackers**

  Good choices include hummus, tahini, fresh butter, nut spreads (Brazil, almond, cashew, natural peanut paste etc.), fresh avocado, pesto sauce, babaganoush, salsa, tomato paste, olive paste and aioli. Make sure that the spreads you buy do not contain hydrogenated vegetable oils or sugar.

  Butter is much healthier than margarine, but it should only be used in moderation and must be very fresh, as rancid butter is oxidized and is bad for the liver.

- **Stocks and flavorings**

  Good choices include miso paste, soy sauce, tamari, all fresh herbs, organic vegetable and organic meat stock cubes, V8 vegetable juice and tomato paste.

- **Oils**

  Cold pressed unrefined olive oil and nut and seed oils are the healthiest - eg. Virgin olive oil, flaxseed oil, sunflower seed oil, macadamia nut oil, walnut oil, grape seed, sesame seed oil etc.

  Coconut oil can be used for Asian stir fries if you want its unique flavor and also for coating vegetables to be roasted. Coconut oil is really quite healthy for the liver and the immune system and is not fattening compared to many other fats.

- **Vinegars**

  The best of all is organic apple cider vinegar made from the whole apple; other healthy vinegars are rice wine vinegar, red wine vinegar and sherry vinegar. Apple cider vinegar helps to heal hemorrhoids and lowers insulin levels.

• **Beverages**

Good choices include organic full cream dairy milk or organic low fat dairy milk (this can be cow's, sheep's or goat's milk), unsweetened soy milk, almond milk, oat milk, rice milk, canned coconut milk (needs diluting with water), water (filtered or purified), freshly made vegetable juices, V8 vegetable juice, canned tomato juice with no added sugar. Tea (all varieties including regular, green or herbal) and caffeinated tea and coffee is fine unless you prefer decaffeinated varieties. Coffee is allowed, as it comes from a natural source – the coffee bean. Ground unprocessed coffee is healthier than instant coffee. Do not drink more than 2 - 3 cups of strong coffee daily.

• **Herbs and Spices**

These are generally good for the liver - good choices include jalapeno pepper, celery seed, celery leaf, peppercorns, chervil leaf, star anise, aniseed, chilli, ginger, coriander (cilantro) leaf, coriander seed, curry, cayenne, bay leaves, caraway seed, lemongrass, thyme, marjoram, mustard seed, turmeric, basil, parsley, paprika, nutmeg, lemon zest, dill leaf, thyme, oregano, sage, garlic, cloves, chives, fenugreek, cardamom, poppy and sesame seeds, horseradish, wasabi, mace, stevia, cloves, cassia, pimento, cumin seed, galangal, cinnamon, organic vanilla essence, saffron, rosemary, mint, fennel leaf and seed, green tea and others if they are natural.

These herbs and spices are especially helpful because they speed up the detoxification process inside the liver cells. Thus, they are cleansing and fat-burning foods.

- **Seaweeds**

  Seaweeds or sea vegetables are very healthy and are eaten in huge amounts by some Asian cultures. Some popular culinary varieties include arame, wakame, nori, dulse and kombu. Seaweeds are high in the health-promoting minerals iodine and calcium.

- **Sweeteners**

  The naturally sweet herb stevia is the best sweetener of all and is 300 times sweeter than sugar; thus only tiny amounts are needed. Stevia extract is available in the form of powder, tablets and drops. You can also grow your own stevia plant and use the leaves to sweeten stir fry dishes, desserts and drinks.

  Sugar alcohols such as xylitol and erythritol are better than sugar, as they have far fewer calories and carbohydrates than sugar. Sugar and honey will spike the blood sugar levels and should be avoided in tea and coffee. For more information on natural sweeteners see page 39.

In general in those with a fatty liver it is best to minimize the intake of foods that are made from grains, especially if the grains are combined with sugar and/or hydrogenated vegetable oils.

In my patients with a moderate to very fatty liver and/or type 2 diabetes, I find it is much more effective if they avoid ALL GRAINS AND SUGAR until their problem is under control; this may vary from 3 months to 12 months.

In those who find that their weight will not budge an ounce, it is also effective to choose a grain free and sugar free diet for at least 3 months.

In those who find it impossible to lose weight, the elimination of ALL grains (wheat, rye, barley, oats, rice, corn) and products made from them, often make it possible to kick start the fat-burning process. In my type 2 diabetic patients I have found that the total elimination of all grains and sugar from the diet often reverses the diabetes.

Basics of shopping

Try to support local farmers and producers, not only to help your local community but also to increase your chances of getting uncontaminated food and fresh food. Ideally find a local grower of organic fruits and vegetables and you may be able to have these foods delivered fresh to your home.

I have noticed that when I buy fruits and vegetables from a local green grocer, or from a side of the road grower/vendor, that the produce is usually fresher and lasts longer. It also tastes so much better than many supermarket or imported vegetables.

Fruits and vegetables from the large supermarkets can look good or even "perfect" but once they have been in your kitchen for 2 to 3 days, they start to deteriorate if their flesh is unhealthy. They start to change color and become contaminated with fungus and bacteria.

Fruits and vegetables from large supermarkets, especially if imported, may have several drawbacks; they may –

- be gas ripened
- have traveled huge distances
- have been kept for long periods in very cold storage
- have been injected with preservatives and colorings

A pale spongy enlarged tomato has far fewer nutrients than a deep red smaller firmer tomato. So do your own research and find a local source of good quality fruits and vegetables.

Buy the fruits and vegetables that are in season – apples in the fall, stone fruit in the summer, asparagus in the spring, cabbage and citrus fruits in the winter etc.

Fresh produce is firm and crisp, whereas older produce is limp and drier.

Storage of produce

- Store garlic, uncut pumpkin, onions and potatoes in a dry place and not in the fridge

- Store mushrooms in paper bags in the fridge

- Store most vegetables – for example broccoli, cabbage, bell peppers (capsicum), courgettes (zucchini), carrots, beets, cut pumpkin, eggplant, leeks etc. - in the vegetable crisper of the fridge

- Store citrus fruits, bananas, pears, stone fruits, apples and unripe avocadoes in a large bowl in a cool well-ventilated part of the kitchen

- Store berries of all varieties in the fridge; they can also be frozen

- Store fresh herbs in a sealed plastic bag in the fridge and they will last for up to a week

- Store dried herbs in sealed glass jars in a cool dark cupboard.

CHAPTER ELEVEN

Healthy Sample Menus for Fatty Liver

Breakfast ideas for one person

One bowl approx 9 oz (250g) of plain (unflavored) full fat or low fat acidophilus yoghurt with 1 - 2 pieces of fresh fruit; if desired use a pinch of stevia powder to sweeten or two tablespoons of Synd-X Slimming Protein Powder

Or

Onc bowl cooked fruit with 4 tablespoons plain unflavored yoghurt; if desired use a pinch of stevia powder to sweeten or two tablespoons of Synd-X Slimming Protein Powder

Or

One bowl Low Carb High Fiber muesli with milk and one piece fresh fruit– see recipe page 124

Or

No Grain High Protein Cereal with milk and one piece fresh fruit – see recipe page 125

Or

Two to four eggs - poached, hard boiled, scrambled, fried with a little cold pressed oil, or as a vegetable omelette or frittata – see recipe page 127.

If desired, accompany with one raw vegetable juice

Or

Two or three lean lamb loin chops grilled or one piece of lean steak grilled with grilled vegetables such as tomatoes, eggplant, onions and mushrooms

Or

One glass 7 - 10 oz (200 - 300mls) of Protein Powder Smoothie Milk Shake (see recipe page 123)

Or

Two pieces of fresh fruit or one bowl of fresh fruit salad with 1.8 - 3.5 oz (50 - 100g) of cheese. Note: apples, kiwi fruit, oranges, cantaloupe, honeydew melon, watermelon, paw paw, pineapple (not canned), passionfruit, persimmons, grapefruit, stone fruits and berries of all types are the most slimming of all fruits

Or

Fresh fruit salad with one handful of raw nuts and seeds or 2 tbsp of LSA. Sprinkle the fruit with 1 - 2 tbsp of Synd-X Slimming Protein Powder

Or

Grilled vegetables such as tomatoes, aubergine (eggplant), courgettes (zucchini) and mushrooms with 1.8 - 3.5 oz (50 - 100g) of melted cheese on top

Or

If you are not hungry you can just have a raw vegetable juice with a small handful of raw nuts and seeds

Lunch ideas for one person

Any of our soups (recipe ideas see pages 89 - 100) with 2 Ryvita crackers. Crackers may be spread with a thin layer of butter or spread with hummus or nut spread

Or

Any fresh vegetable salad – (recipe ideas see pages 104 - 120). Salad may be accompanied with 3.5 oz (100g) of cheese or 6.5 oz (185g) can of fish or 1 to 2 grilled chicken drumsticks

Or

Lean fresh grilled steak or 2 lamb chops with a salad (recipe ideas see page 104 - 120) or one cup grilled vegetables

Or

Fish – choose from canned 3.3 or 6.5 oz (95 or 185g can), or fresh fish, grilled or pan fried. Accompany with a fresh garden salad

Or

Red or white meat, seafood or poultry – chopped into bite sized pieces and placed on one or two skewers with vegetable pieces. Skewers can be grilled or barbecued. Serve with a garden salad or raw vegetable juice.

Or

Chicken roasted or grilled 1 - 2 drumsticks or 1 - 2 breasts (eat less if you are not that hungry) – free range organic is much better, with any of our salads (see recipes on page 104 - 120)

Or

One bowl of a legume dish, accompanied with a fresh salad

Or

One bowl approx 9 oz (250g) of plain unflavored full fat or low fat yoghurt with 1 - 2 pieces of fresh fruit and a small handful of raw nuts

Or

Any cooked vegetables (left over from night before) with a fresh vegetable salad and 1.8 oz (50g) of cheese

Or

Egg dish – hard boiled, scrambled or frittata (see recipe on page 127). Hard boiled eggs are nice in salad with avocado and olives. If you are hungry you can eat up to 4 hard boiled eggs – they are not fattening!!

Or

If you are not hungry you can just have a raw vegetable juice with a handful of raw nuts and seeds

Dinner ideas for one person

One plate of stir fry chicken, lamb, beef, seafood or tofu with mixed vegetables

Or

One piece steak or 2 - 3 lean lamb or veal chops grilled or barbequed accompanied with fresh salad and steamed vegetables

Or

One bowl 9 - 17 oz (250 - 500ml) of meat and vegetable casserole

Or

One bowl 9 - 17 oz (250 - 500ml) of chicken and vegetable soup

Or

One bowl 9 - 17 oz (250 - 500ml) of legume and vegetable casserole

Or

One bowl 9 - 17 oz (250 - 500ml) of stir fry beans with vegetables. You can add nuts and seeds to this if desired

Or

Fish - 1 - 2 fillets or one whole fish - grilled, barbequed, steamed, turbo cooked, baked or stuffed. Accompany with cooked vegetables or a fresh salad

Or

Chicken - 1 - 2 drumsticks, or 2 - 3 thigh fillets or 1 - 2 breasts, roasted, grilled or barbequed with roast vegetables

Or

Lean white or red meat, seafood or poultry - chopped into pieces and placed on 2 skewers with vegetable pieces - grill, barbecue or roast. Accompany with fresh garden salad

Or

Egg dishes - 3 egg omelette, or 3 - 4 eggs scrambled or a large slice of frittata accompanied with fresh salad

After Dinner Desserts

These can be eaten if you are still hungry, but choose fresh fruit salad or one of our recipes –see page 140.

CHAPTER TWELVE

· ·

Raw Juicing Can Heal Your Liver

Use raw juices for breakfast or as snacks, or you may use a raw juice as a meal replacement if you are not hungry.

It is best to make your own fresh raw juices with a juice-extracting machine, as bottled juices may contain sugar, have lost enzyme and vitamin content and may have been pasteurized. Alternatively you can buy freshly made raw juices at the many juice bars now available. You can also make a large supply and freeze it immediately.

Generally you need the juice to be comprised of 80% vegetables and 20% fruit, although you may reduce the amount of fruit more, to reduce the carbohydrate content even more. Indeed you do not have to include any fruit in the juice and can make it with vegetables only; generally the fruit is used to improve or vary the taste of the juice. If you use too much fruit in your juice, the higher carbohydrate content may make it harder to lose weight.

Many bottled fruit juices are too high in sugar and some juice bars use a stock base of pasteurized juice, which is lower in vital nutrients than a freshly extracted juice.

Raw vegetable juices are able to speed up the repair of liver damage

Our juice recipes help to repair the liver, stimulate the detoxification pathways and improve the fat burning capability of the liver.

The best juices for the liver are made from such things as green beans, Brussels sprouts, broccoli, purple and green cabbage, parsley, mint, coriander, basil, radish, ginger root, carrot, pears, citrus, apple and beets. You may add a dash of chicory, chives, dandelion leaves, garlic and red onion for extra benefit. For more information and juice recipes and also to learn how you can grow your own dandelion see page 86.

Why Juice?

Most people's fruit and vegetable intake is well below the eight recommended servings daily. Juices are a tasty and efficient way to increase fruit and vegetable intake. Many nutrients, including vitamin C, disappear quickly when vegetables and fruit are cooked or left to sit in the open air and light. Fresh juice contains a full range of healing nutrients, as well as beneficial active enzymes. Combining citrus with other fruits and vegetables delivers a powerful synergistic cocktail of vitamin C, folate, minerals, antioxidants and plant pigments.

Juicing concentrates the protective antioxidants and anti-cancer substances present in fruits and vegetables.

Research has shown that antioxidants are able to prevent, repair and reverse liver damage to a significant degree.

Make fresh juice a regular part of your life

Many people start out juicing with good intentions, but lose interest over time. Most people stop juicing because they run out of time and it becomes too much of an effort. Here are a few tips to take the work out of juicing.

- Choose a time of day when you can enjoy juicing. Juice is lovely in the morning, but if you are too busy in the morning, choose another time! A fresh fruit and vegetable juice is nice in the afternoon when you get home from work, or even after dinner.

- Buy a juicer that is easy to clean. The biggest reason that people stop juicing is that they do not want to clean the juicer. A good juicer takes just 3-4 minutes to clean.

Time yourself, and then consider: How much time is your health worth? You can also try cleaning it immediately after juicing, and then sit down to enjoy your juice. End with the reward.

- Buy a juicer with a large feed chute. This means less chopping. For many fruits and vegetables, you can simply wash and go. Oranges should usually be peeled, and that's it!

- Buy two different juice machines – one with a fast centrifugal chopping bowl and one with a grinder masticator squeezing mechanism. The centrifugal juicers can be purchased cheaply and are time saving for hard vegetables such as carrots, beet, celery, fennel and pumpkin etc. Conversely the grinder masticator juicers have a slower more gentle action suitable for soft produce such as green leafy herbs, citrus fruits, pineapple, pears and tomatoes. The grinder masticator juicers extract more juice from these softer types of produce and do not overheat their nutrients and enzymes.

- Experiment a little with the contents of your fridge. If you do not have all of the ingredients for the juice recipe, then improvise! Citrus juice combines very well with almost any fruit, herb or vegetable.

- Keep the juicer on the counter. It may be tempting to hide it away, but if you store the juicer where you will see it every day, you are more likely to use it every day.

- Make a whole week's supply of juice at one time – as soon as it is made, pour it into glass jars, leave a one inch space at the top of the jar, put the lid on the jars, and place them in the freezer. If you freeze the juice immediately, it will preserve and retain all the vitamins, enzymes and other healing nutrients perfectly for months.

You need around 6.8oz (200mls) of juice daily, which is not a lot when you think about it. I freeze a week's supply of my juice and this is a great time-saving tip!

Vitamin C and the liver

I think that vitamin C is the most beneficial vitamin for the liver because it is such a powerful protective and healing antioxidant. Vitamin C is able to neutralize the dangerous free radicals that are produced in the liver by incorrect foods, certain drugs and during the liver's detoxification of toxic chemicals. We need to obtain a lot of vitamin C from our diet every day, especially if we have a liver problem and the recommended daily allowance of 30 - 100mg is very inadequate. The work of Nobel Prize winner Linus Pauling showed that many people need thousands of milligrams of vitamin C everyday.

All fresh fruits and vegetables contain vitamin C, but citrus is one of the best. With 62 mg per orange, citrus beats out pineapple, peaches and apples.

Low carbohydrate (carb) is good for fatty liver

The World Health Organization recognizes that fruits and vegetables are important for the prevention of liver disease and obesity. This is because fruit and vegetables are high in nutrients, but low in carbohydrate and fat. Citrus fruits are the perfect example. Lemons, limes and grapefruit have the lowest carbohydrate content of any fruit.

FRUIT	*Grams of carbs per serving*
Lime	0.6
Lemon	1.8
Grapefruit	4.8
Cantaloupe	7.5
Kiwifruit	7.8
Orange	9.5
Grapes	11.9
Mango	18.9
Apple	20.0
Banana	27.9

Types of carbohydrate in fruits

There is another reason why citrus is suitable for people watching their carbohydrate intake. Fruit sugar, or fructose, is the main carbohydrate in citrus fruit. Fructose acts very differently in the body compared to refined sugar (glucose) or starch. Fructose enters the blood stream slowly, and, because in fruit it is contained in a lot of water, citrus has a low glycaemic index. Oranges, grapefruit, lemons and limes are good foods for diabetics who need to maintain a stable blood sugar, and for people trying to lose weight.

Include some citrus peel!

Flavonoids are very powerful anti-inflammatory nutrients found in citrus fruits. While appreciable amounts of the healing flavonoids are found in the juice itself, the highest concentration of flavonoids is located in the peel and the white pith just below the peel. Include a little bit of orange peel or zest in your diet to significantly increase your daily flavonoid intake.

Citrus peel has the highest concentration of the super-flavonoids, such as tangeretin and limonene. These phytochemicals are powerful anti-inflammatory and healing antioxidants.

New research shows that these phytochemicals are effective for –

- Improving liver function
- Lowering cholesterol
- Dissolving gallstones
- Preventing cancer

Although citrus peel is strong tasting, and has been traditionally removed before juicing, it is possible to use some of the peel in your juices. When the peel is mixed with other things such as carrots, apples, pineapple etc, the taste is deliciously different.

Start slowly by leaving ¼ of the orange unpeeled. Be sure to also leave plenty of the white pith directly below the peel, because it is also a major source of flavonoids and is not bitter. Pass the peel and pith through the juicer with the other produce to get a creamy, frothy juice.

RAW JUICE RECIPES

If the juices are too strong and/or upset your stomach, taste unpleasant or give you diarrhea, you should dilute them with plenty of water, extra celery or eliminate or reduce the amounts of the ingredients which upset you.

You can vary the ingredients and their amounts to give you more enjoyment and variety.

Most of these recipes will produce 1 - 2 cups of juice.

JUICES FOR THE LIVER AND GALLSTONES
Morning Lemon Cleanse

½ -1 lemon, freshly squeezed
8 oz (250ml) warm water

Fresh lemon juice contains the phytochemical limonene, which improves liver function, and is used in Japan to dissolve gallstones.

Morning is the best time for lemon juice because it is also a natural liver decongestant and gentle laxative.

Liver Cleansing Juice

½ lemon with some peel
2 apples, unpeeled
2 dandelion or 2 arugula or 2 cabbage leaves
½ cup broccoli florets, chopped
1 clove garlic or ¼ red onion (can use less if desired)
½ cup parsley

This is a strong mixture and may be diluted with 1 cup water, extra celery or dandelion root tea.

Fatty Liver Juice

½ *whole lemon or grapefruit, peeled*
2 carrots, peeled
1 clove garlic or ¼ *red onion (optional or use less if it is too strong)*
½ *inch (1cm) slice fennel*
¼ *beet, peeled*
2 dandelion or 2 arugula or 2 cabbage leaves

Apples or celery may be added to improve the taste.

Liver Healing Juice

1 orange, peeled
2 carrots, peeled
1 apple with skin
1 clove garlic or 1 small spring onion (may use less or avoid if you have a sensitive stomach)
½ *beet, peeled and tops*
½ *cup watercress*

Gallstone Dissolving Juice

½ *lemon with some peel and pith*
2 cabbage or 2 dandelion or 2 arugula or 2 baby spinach leaves
¼ *beet, peeled*
1 large apple, unpeeled
2 Brussels sprouts
1 large tomato
¼ *inch (*½ *cm) ginger root*

If you have gallstones, start slowly with this juice because it is designed to shrink and gradually dissolve gallstones. You can dilute it with water, extra apples or celery or dandelion root tea.
Aim to drink 70 - 105 oz (2 - 3 liters) of water per day.

SYNDROME X AND DIABETES

Fatty liver is associated with a much higher risk of Syndrome X and diabetes.

Syndrome X can be most easily described as a pre-diabetic condition because in those with Syndrome X there is impairment of the ability of the body to handle sugar.

Unlike Type 1 diabetics, who are dependent on insulin injections, Type 2 diabetics usually have insulin levels that are normal or high. Their bodies do not respond to the insulin effectively anymore and this is known as insulin resistance

In the early to medium stages,
Type 2 diabetes is reversible.

The best approach to achieve this includes -

- A low carbohydrate eating plan as contained in this book
- Supplements to improve the function of insulin – such as Magnesium, Glicemic Balance, cinammon, turmeric, fenugreek and chromium
- A liver tonic and a diet plentiful in raw vegetables to improve the liver function

JUICES FOR SYNDROME X OR TYPE 2 DIABETES

The juice recipes below are suitable for those with Syndrome X or Type 2 diabetes.

Generally speaking, Type 1 diabetics are better to use the whole fruit or vegetable, rather than juice, although there are exceptions.

Diabetes and Syndrome X Juice

½ grapefruit, peeled but with pith left on
¼ bitter melon peeled (if available, otherwise leave out)
2 carrots, peeled
2 dandelion leaves or 2 cabbage leaves

1 spring onion or ½ clove garlic
½ cup green beans
¼ cup fennel

Mix with ½ tsp fenugreek powder steeped for 20 minutes in ¼ cup hot water

Cholesterol-lowering Juice

2 oranges or tangerines, with some peel and white pith
1 grapefruit, peeled
1 tomato
1 clove garlic or ¼ red onion (reduce amounts if stomach is sensitive)
2 cabbage leaves or 2 dandelion or 2 arugula or 2 baby spinach leaves
1 radish, unpeeled with tops

WEIGHT LOSS JUICE RECIPES FOR FATTY LIVER
Low Carbohydrate

Citrus is actually lower in carbohydrates than many vegetables, and it has a low glycaemic index.

Low Carbohydrate Slimming Juice

1 orange with ¼ peel and pith left on
2 sticks celery
½ cucumber, peeled
½ cup green beans
2 sprigs parsley

Orange is naturally low in sugar.

Cucumber, celery and parsley are natural diuretics and reduce cellulite.

Green beans lower insulin and blood sugar levels.

Fat burning Juice

1 orange, peeled
1 grapefruit, peeled
1 carrot, peeled
2 stalks celery with leaves removed
½ inch (1cm) slice ginger root
1 red radish
Pinch cayenne

Dilute 50% with green tea if desired.

> **Those with a fatty liver have a slow metabolism that stores fat.**
>
> **They need to eat foods that will increase the rate that food energy is dissipated as heat. These foods are known as thermogenic foods.**

Research shows that the vitamins and phytochemicals in raw fruits and vegetables work together to stimulate faster metabolism and increase fat burning.

Orange, limes, lemons and grapefruit increase thermogenesis.

Celery is a natural diuretic.

Ginger, radish and cayenne increase basal metabolic rate.

Green tea contains catechin and natural caffeine, which increase the metabolic rate.

How to grow your own dandelion

Dandelion is a herb with proven ability to heal and revitalize the liver. In many countries dandelion is a weed which grows abundantly on roadsides, fields and gardens, but when grown under controlled conditions it is a very useful herb.

There are specialized herb nurseries where you can purchase a cultivated dandelion plant or you can lift a small dandelion plant from a garden and plant it in a pot.

Look after your plant until new leaves grow, and use only the new leaves in your salads and juices. When the plant is stable, remove all the old original leaves; you now have a cultivated dandelion plant and can use the leaves as you would from any other culinary/medicinal herb. Two plants should be sufficient for your juicing needs.

It is important to remove any flower heads as they appear from your plant because if allowed to seed you will have a problem with weeds.

If you run out of dandelion, other healing leaves that can be juiced or added to salads are radish, turnip and beet leaves, silver beet and spinach.

CHAPTER THIRTEEN

Healthy Liver Recipes

Basics of healthy cooking

Preferred methods of cooking

- A good way to preserve the nutrients in food is by using a pressure cooker
- Steam, grill, or stir-fry as first preference, and use only cold pressed oils, not cheap vegetable oils
- Roasting, braising and baking are healthy ways to cook provided you don't use too much fat
- Braise vegetables in the oven, or on top of the stove, in as little liquid as possible
- Steam vegetables over the top of water or cook them gently in a small amount of water

Least healthy ways of cooking

- Avoid or minimize using microwave ovens for cooking or re-heating meals
- Never cook or reheat food in a plastic container in a microwave oven
- Avoid overcooking vegetables – cook only until they are al dente
- Avoid shallow or deep frying food, especially at high temperatures, as these methods use a lot of fat and damage the fat
- Avoid boiling vegetables, as you will lose most of the nutrients in the water

Note: if using a non-stick pan it is safer to avoid Teflon coated pans. There is a new pan designed in Belgium called GREENPAN and its THERMOLON non-stick coating is PTFE-free, heat resistant and releases no toxic fumes – visit www.green-pan.com

LIVER HEALTHY SOUP RECIPES

I am a great believer in the use of healthy soups to heal and regenerate the liver.

The soup recipes we have included are most beneficial for those with fatty liver because –

- They contain healthy and cleansing ingredients, antioxidants and minerals
- They are light and easily digested and do not overload the liver or intestines
- They can be used as a complete meal when combined with a fresh salad

You can make up a large amount of the soup using fresh ingredients and the soup can be stored in the freezer for weeks. This makes it easy for you to have a liver cleansing soup everyday, or just when you feel like it for a snack.

I advise you not to reheat any meals with a microwave oven – after your fine efforts to make the soup, why would you want to damage the structure of the nutrients with microwave radiation?

Dr. Cabot's Liver Healing Soup Recipe

Serves 6 - 8

8 cups water

miso and/or tamari to taste

3 tablespoons of cold pressed olive oil

2 sweet potatoes, chopped

3 tomatoes, chopped

2 carrots, chopped

2 leeks, washed and sliced

1 bunch spinach (fresh or frozen), chopped

2 stalks of celery (including the tops), chopped

2 large brown onions, chopped

1 inch (2.5cm) finely chopped and peeled ginger root

2 cloves garlic, minced (optional)

1 bunch sliced kale or beet greens

1 cup cooked beans or lentils

Add small amounts of celery seed, turmeric, pepper and miso (or tamari) to taste

optional added extra ingredients:

2 - 3 fresh artichoke hearts

2 cups shiitake mushrooms fresh or reconstituted sliced

1 whole reishi mushroom (remove when cooked)

¼ cup arame or wakame seaweed chopped

Although these 4 ingredients are traditionally very good for the liver and the immune system, not everyone likes these things, so if they really do not appeal to you, leave some or all of them out.

In a large saucepan add the oil and bring to a moderate to high heat. Add the celery (plus tops), ginger root, turmeric, tomato, potato, carrots, onions, celery seed and garlic and some pepper.

Stir continuously so the vegetables do not stick to the bottom. When the vegetables begin to brown, carefully add the water with miso/tamari to taste. Bring to the boil. Reduce the heat to a simmer. Add the lentils/beans and stir. If using these, add the seaweed, mushrooms and artichoke hearts. Simmer for about 2 hours.

Add the kale and beet greens 15 minutes before you serve. If present, remove the reishi mushrooms.

Stir in the miso/tamari to taste.

Serve alone or with a side salad and one slice crusty wholemeal bread.

Chickpea Soup

Serves 4 - 6

2 cloves garlic, chopped
14 oz (400g) can chopped tomatoes
1 tbsp tomato paste
14 oz (400g) can chickpeas, drained
1 tbsp finely chopped cilantro (coriander) leaves
1 tsp curry powder
1 tsp cumin spice
2 tbsp chopped mushrooms
2 tbsp cold pressed olive oil
1 bell pepper (capsicum), chopped
½ tsp mustard seeds
4 cups vegetable stock or water and vegetable stock cube
Salt and freshly ground pepper to taste

Heat oil on medium heat in a large saucepan. Add the garlic, onion, mustard seeds, and curry powder and stir for several minutes.

Add the bell pepper, chopped mushrooms, chopped tomatoes, tomato paste, stock or water, and simmer for 5 minutes. Add the drained chickpeas into the soup and simmer for 10 minutes. Season with salt and pepper, and stir in cilantro just before serving.

If desired, grate some Parmesan cheese over the top.

Lamb and Vegetable soup

Serves 6

2½ pints (1.5 liters) water
1 vegetable stock cube
1 lamb or beef stock cube
2 tbsp olive oil
2.2lb (1kg) lamb chops or lamb necks, remove excess fat
2 oz (55g) lentils
2 carrots, chopped
1 parsnip, diced
1 large onion, chopped
2 bay leaves
½ cup V8 vegetable juice
bouquet garni
2 sticks celery with tops, chopped
1 leek washed thoroughly and chopped
1 tablespoon fresh parsley chopped, to garnish

Brown the trimmed meat in olive oil in a large saucepan place water and stock cubes, lentils and bay leaves bring to the boil and simmer for ½ hour.

Cut meat into bite sized pieces - preserving some bone for more flavor. Brown onions in oil and add to meat pieces. Add all other ingredients to meat. Pour lentils and stock on top, cover and simmer gently for 1½ hours. Remove bouquet garni and bay leaves.

Serve garnished with parsley.

Tomato Soup

Serves 6 - 8

1 - 2 tbsp cold-pressed virgin olive oil
1 - 3 garlic cloves, minced (optional)
4 onions, diced
2 celery stalks with leaves, sliced
6 - 8 whole fresh tomatoes – chopped finely
1 cup V8 vegetable juice (spicy or regular)
4 cups vegetable stock or 4 cups water with 1-2 organic vegetable stock cubes or ½ cup tamari
2 tbsp tomato paste
1 handful basil, finely chopped
1 tbsp fresh thyme, finely chopped
1 handful fresh parsley, finely chopped
2 bay leaves
1 dstspn freshly chopped or dried oregano
Pinch sea salt
½ cup finely chopped fresh parsley

Heat the oil in a wok, add the garlic and onion and saute for 5 minutes. Add the celery and sauté for 3 minutes. Add the fresh tomatoes and all the herbs (except for half the parsley). Sauté for 3 minutes. Add all the liquids.

Cook slowly with lid on for 20 minutes over low heat. Add tomato paste and stir well, cook covered for another 15 minutes.

If you desire a thicker soup, use 2 tbsp potato starch or corn flour or rice flour – make into a thick paste with any milk, then add more milk to thin the paste. With wooden spoon, one spoon at a time, stir into the soup to avoid lumps. Cover pot and cook for another 10 minutes.

Garnish with half the parsley and grated parmesan cheese just prior to serving.

Asparagus Soup

Serves 6

1 ½ lbs (675g) fresh green asparagus
2 ½ tbsp coriander seeds, crushed
1 ¾ pints (28oz or 1 liter) chicken or vegetable stock
1 red (Spanish) onion, peeled & chopped
1 lemon – squeezed
sea salt & pepper
2 tbsp cold pressed olive oil
parmesan cheese grated

Heat oil in large saucepan, add the onion and sauté for 3 minutes. Cut the tips off the asparagus and store in fridge. Chop the rest of the asparagus and put them and the coriander seeds in the saucepan. Cover the saucepan and heat for 5 minutes, then add the stock and 13.6oz (400 ml) water. Simmer gently on low heat for 10 to 15 minutes until asparagus is tender. Puree the soup in a blender and then pass through a sieve. Leave to cool and cover and chill. Season with salt, pepper and some lemon juice to your liking and then chill again. Steam the stored asparagus tips until just tender. Serve the soup over the tops of the asparagus tips in chilled small bowls. Sprinkle over parmesan cheese.

NOTES - Vegetable soups

You may use any vegetables of your choice and use miso, tamari or vegetable stock cubes to flavor. You can add beans, chickpeas and lentils if desired to provide extra protein, fiber and phyto-estrogens, which have an anti-cancer effect.

The Happy Liver Soup

Serves 4

½ cup red lentils and 1 cup brown lentils
2 tsp soy sauce
1 tbsp dried basil or handful of fresh basil, finely chopped
1 tsp dried oregano
1 tsp dried thyme
½ tsp chilli powder (optional)
1 sprig fresh rosemary finely chopped from the stalk
1 handful fresh parsley, chopped
2 tbsp cold-pressed virgin olive oil
1 large leek, chopped and well washed
2 medium size brown onions finely chopped
2 sticks celery with leaves finely chopped
2 tomatoes, finely chopped
2 carrots, chopped
6 cups pure water
1 cup V8 vegetable juice
½ organic vegetable stock cube
2 bay leaves
sea salt, ground black pepper

Add oil to pan and on low heat, gently fry the lentils for 2 minutes. Add onion, garlic and tomatoes and heat for 3 minutes, add all herbs (except for half the parsley) and cook 2 minutes while stirring. Add all the liquids, bay leaves and stock cubes - gently simmer for 10 minutes with lid on.

Add the leek, carrot and celery. Cook on low heat for 1 hour, stirring the pot occasionally.

Garnish with parsley and grated parmesan to serve.

Pumpkin Soup

Serves 8

2 small squash (butternut pumpkin), diced
3 cups of a dark orange colored pumpkin, diced
2 onions, diced
2 garlic cloves, minced
2 stalks celery with leaves, chopped
2 carrots, chopped
6 cups vegetable stock or Campbell's All Natural Stock
2 tbsp olive oil
¼ bunch fresh basil
2 tbsp soy sauce or Tamari
Pinch sea salt
Freshly ground black pepper
3 bay leaves
¼ bunch flat-leaf parsley, chopped
1 cup milk

In a soup pot add oil, onions and garlic and fry for 2 minutes. Add all herbs and tamari and stir for 2 minutes. Add all the liquids to the pot. Add in all the vegetables including the pumpkin. Add soy sauce, salt, pepper, bay leaves and parsley. Bring to a boil, reduce heat and simmer on a very low heat for 1 hour. Allow to cool, remove bay leaves and blend soup in a blender or food processor until smooth. Add milk in the blender last, and use more if mixture is too thick.

Garnish with fresh parsley and a dollop of full cream yoghurt with some grated nutmeg on top of soup (you can grate your own nutmeg – simply delicious!)

Traditional Chicken Soup

Serves 4 - 6

You can purchase ready made chicken stock (organic is preferable) or make your own stock

To make the stock:
1 free-range chicken or chicken thighs (with bones) and breasts (skin removed)
2 cups celery tops chopped
2 bay leaves
1 large brown onion
2 garlic cloves

Simmer slowly for 90 minutes under cover, the whole chicken or chicken parts, with the bay leaves, onion, celery tops, parsley and garlic cloves in approx 50oz (1.5 liters) of water. Strain the liquid into a soup pot. Keep the chicken and the stock in the refrigerator overnight.

To make the soup:
2 large onions, diced
2 carrots, finely chopped
½ bunch fresh basil
3 stalks celery with leaves, finely chopped
1 cup flat-leaf parsley, chopped
2 small parsnip, finely chopped
2 cups V8 vegetable juice (optional)
2 small turnip, finely chopped
2 bay leaves
Sea salt to taste
Freshly ground black pepper

Gently fry the onions in oil. Take the chicken from refrigerator and cut off all chicken meat into cubes. Keep some of the large bones aside. Skim fat from top of stock.
In a large soup pot place stock, chicken pieces and bones. Simmer 5 minutes with lid on.
Finely chop all vegetables and herbs and add to the pot with the onion. Cover and simmer for approximately 2 hours.
Remove bay leaves and chicken bones.
Season with sea salt and black pepper to taste.

Fish and Spinach Soup

Serves 4

8 spinach leaves, washed, stems removed, finely chopped
1 tbsp olive oil
27 oz (800ml) chicken stock or fish stock
7 oz (200g) crushed tomatoes
2 sticks celery
1 red onion, chopped
1 clove garlic, crushed
2 courgettes (zucchini), diced
¼ fresh fennel bulb, chopped (optional)
1 tsp grated ginger
2 tbsp tamari sauce
9oz (250g) white fish fillets, diced
salt and pepper

Heat a saucepan over low heat, add olive oil, garlic and onion and cook for 3 minutes. Add stock and tomatoes and bring to boil, add fennel, ginger, courgettes and celery. Cover and simmer for 5 minutes. Add fish, tamari, spinach, salt, pepper and stir - cook for 10 minutes or until fish flakes easily with a fork.

Seafood Soup

Serves 6 - 8

Any fish and/or shell fish can be used in this soup
2 sticks celery, with some leaves left on, sliced
2 large potatoes, chopped – the potatoes can be left out if you want a very low carb variety of this soup
1 whole chilli, seeded, sliced (optional)
5 cups stock, (fish or vegetable) or 5 cups water with 1 - 2 organic vegetable stock cubes
¾ cup white wine
4.4 lb (2 kg) fish and/or shellfish prepared

2 onions, chopped
2 cloves garlic, half thinly sliced, half crushed
6 medium ripe chopped tomatoes
½ bunch fresh dill, chopped
½ bunch parsley, chopped
½ bunch cilantro (coriander), chopped
1 lemon juiced
3 tbsp cold pressed olive oil
sea salt and ground black pepper

Brown the onion, thinly sliced garlic and celery in oil for 2 minutes. Add the crushed garlic and chilli, cook for 1 minute. Add potatoes, stir constantly till slightly golden. Pour in stock and lemon juice. Simmer until potatoes are tender then add fish, shellfish, tomatoes, all the herbs and seasonings. Cook on low heat until seafood is tender.
Serve with fresh green salad.

Minestrone Soup
Serves 4
2 large brown onions, peeled
½ bunch of fresh basil
1 tsp chilli powder or 1 tsp mild paprika
¼ bunch fresh cilantro (coriander)
½ bunch of flat-leaf parsley, finely chopped
1 sprig fresh rosemary, chopped off stalk
1 large can V8 vegetable juice or 6 cups Vegetable Stock
2 tbsp soy sauce
2 vegetable stock cubes (free of MSG)
13 oz (370g) canned or 6 fresh tomatoes
½ cup brown lentils
1 cup red kidney beans
½ cup navy beans
½ cup lima beans

4 bay leaves
2 garlic cloves (optional)
2 stalks celery with leaves, finely chopped
2 carrots, finely chopped
1 parsnip, finely chopped
1 small turnip, finely chopped
1 leek, chopped finely
2 tbsp cold pressed olive oil
Freshly ground black pepper to taste

Fry the onions and garlic in a pan in oil for 2 minutes, put all herbs in a food processor and blend until finely chopped.

In a large soup pot place the vegetable stock or V8 juice, soy sauce, 1 cup hot water, and stock cubes mixed with 1 cup warm water. Stir and add the onion, garlic and herb mix from the blender into pot. Place the tomatoes in the food processor and blend, add to soup pot.

Add the lentils, and all chopped vegetables and bay leaves to the pot. Cover and cook slowly on low heat for 60 minutes stirring occasionally, season with black pepper if desired.

Add all the beans and cook for another 30 minutes on low heat. Remove the bay leaves.

Buy organic canned beans already cooked and rinse before adding to pot.

Alternatively to prepare beans: soak dried beans in water for 4 hours. Drain.

Using fresh water with a slice of lemon, cook the beans for approximately 45 - 60 minutes until tender.

Salad Dressings and Dips

You may be surprised to learn that many of the pre-made bottled salad dressings in supermarkets are very unhealthy for those with a fatty liver.

When you look on their labels you see ingredients such as cheap refined vegetable oil and sugar or dextrose and preservatives; these are high in carbohydrates.

On this program you will be eating a lot of salads, so it's important to use healthy salad dressings. You can also buy healthy salad dressings that are made with cold pressed oils and are free of sugar, but you need to read the labels.

Avocado Spread / Dip

1 large ripe avocado, peeled
½ tsp finely grated lemon rind
1 clove garlic, crushed
1 cup plain yoghurt
1 tbsp cold pressed olive oil
½ lemon, juiced
1 tsp honey
¼ cup red onion, finely chopped
2 tsp parsley, finely chopped
salt and pepper

Place all ingredients (except onion and parsley) in blender and blend until smooth. Stir in onion and parsley.

Mint Dressing

¼ cup cold pressed olive oil
1 tbsp fresh mint, chopped
½ cup lemon or orange juice freshly squeezed
½ cup plain yoghurt
1 tsp honey (optional)

Mix and chill to use the same day.

Yoghurt Salad Dressing or Dip

1 cup plain yoghurt
1 tbsp fresh basil, chopped
1 tbsp fresh parsley, chopped
1 tbsp fresh chives, chopped
1 tbsp tomato paste
1 tsp Dijon mustard
1 garlic clove, minced
½ tsp cracked black pepper

Combine all ingredients and mix. Chill in refrigerator for 2 hours to blend flavors. Serve garnished with fresh parsley.

Tamari Dressing

½ cup cold pressed olive oil
½ cup Balsamic vinegar or freshly squeezed lemon juice
1 dstpn tamari
1 tsp honey (optional)
1 tbsp fresh basil chopped

Put all ingredients into a jar, shake well. Store in refrigerator.

Hummus Dressing

3 tbsp hummus (see recipe page 121)
1 tbsp tahini
1 lemon, freshly squeezed
1 clove garlic, minced
1 tbsp cold pressed olive oil

Place in blender and bend until smooth. Pour into a jar and store in refrigerator.

Sesame Oil Dressing

¼ cup cold pressed sesame oil
¼ cup cold pressed olive oil
1 tsp sesame seeds, dry roasted
1 tsp honey
1 tsp fresh garlic, minced
1 tsp fresh coriander, chopped
½ cup fresh squeezed lemon juice
½ tsp dried cumin

Put all ingredients, except the seeds, into a jar and shake well. Store dressing in refrigerator. Store seeds in a glass jar, as they are sprinkled over salad when serving.

Mustard Dressing

1 tsp honey
2 tsp grainy mustard
2 tbsp cold pressed olive oil
1 lemon, juiced
1 tbsp apple cider vinegar

Mix together well in a jar and store in refrigerator.

Basic Mayonnaise

2 egg yolks
¼ tsp pepper
2 tbsp apple cider vinegar
1 tsp dry mustard
½ tsp sea salt
2 tbsp freshly squeezed lemon juice
¼ tsp paprika
½ cup cold pressed virgin olive oil
1 tsp honey

Put egg yolks into a bowl, add mustard, salt, honey, pepper, paprika and beat together all ingredients thoroughly.

Add 2 tbsp vinegar slowly while stirring then add the oil drop by drop.

Stir hard with a wooden spoon until mayonnaise is thick and smooth.

Add lemon juice gradually and then beat vigorously.

This basic recipe can be varied by adding other flavors to it. Try adding the following to 4 oz (115mls) of basic mayonnaise recipe:

Curry Mayo - blend 2 tsp curry powder with 2 tbsp milk and stir into mayo.

Green Mayo - just add very finely chopped fresh herbs of choice.

Horseradish Mayo - blend 1 tbsp horseradish with mayo.

Lemon Mayo - add the grated rind (zest) of 1 lemon and ½ its juice to mayo.

Spiced Mayo - add some grated nutmeg and a few drops of Worcestershire sauce to mayo.

Salads

Watercress and Fennel Cleansing Salad

This salad is great for those with a sluggish gall bladder, gallstones and/or fatty liver. It promotes the flow of bile and improves digestion.

Serves 2

1 small bunch watercress, washed and chopped
1 large fennel bulb, washed and thinly sliced

1 handful fresh parsley, washed, dried and chopped finely
½ lemon thinly sliced
1 tbsp fresh squeezed lemon juice
sea salt and black pepper

You may add some fresh dandelion leaves, washed and chopped if you have them!

Mix together the parsley, watercress and fennel and season with lemon juice and salt and pepper. Cut each lemon slice into small segments and add to the salad.

Use one of our lovely salad dressings or just cold pressed oil and lemon juice.

Beetroot Salad - Moroccan Style

Serves 4

9 oz (250g) beets, steamed with skins removed
3 tbsp fresh coriander leaves, chopped
2 tbsp fresh mint leaves, chopped
1 tsp coriander seeds, roasted and ground or 1 tsp dried coriander spice
3 tbsp red onion, chopped finely
4 tbsp virgin cold pressed olive oil
1 tbsp walnut or macadamia oil
2 lemons freshly squeezed – use the juice
½ cup lightly roasted walnuts, chopped
4 young beet leaves
Pepper and sea salt to taste

While the beets are warm, chop them into bite-sized chunks, mix with ground coriander, onion and herbs.

Whisk the oils and lemon juice together in a bowl, season with salt and pepper.

Toss all ingredients throughout the dressing.

Spinach Salad

Serves 4

1 bunch small leaf spinach
4 tbsp sesame seeds
2 tbsp cold-pressed virgin olive oil or macadamia oil
1 tbsp lemon juice freshly squeezed
1 tsp soy sauce
A dash of Tabasco or sambal olek (chilli paste) - optional
9 oz (260g) can water chestnuts, drained and sliced
8 button mushrooms, sliced

Remove the spinach stems, wash thoroughly then dry in a clean cloth or paper towel. Place in the refrigerator with the cloth to crisp.

Toast the sesame seeds in a pan over moderate heat, shaking constantly. Remove from the pan and let cool. Mix the oil, lemon juice, soy sauce, and Tabasco as dressing.

Place the torn spinach leaves in a salad bowl and coat with the dressing. Then add the chestnuts and mushrooms on top of the leaves and sprinkle with toasted sesame seeds.

Tomato and Onion Salad

Serves 4

19 oz (500g) firm but ripe tomatoes, thinly sliced
4 scallions / green onions, finely sliced or ½ finely chopped red onion
1 cup fresh basil finely chopped
Grated zest of 1 lemon
1 tbsp freshly squeezed lemon juice
2 tbsp cold-pressed virgin olive oil
Freshly ground black pepper and sea salt
½ teaspoon honey

Arrange the tomato slices in a shallow bowl, sprinkle with the lemon zest and pepper.

Dressing; beat lemon juice with oil, sea salt, and honey. Place onions and basil over tomatoes, drizzle the dressing over the lot and refrigerate for 1 hour before serving.

Sprouts Galore Salad

Serves 4 - 6

8 scallions / green onions, cut diagonally

12 button mushrooms, sliced thinly

1 red apple, cored and cut into thin slices

2 tomatoes, diced

4 stalks celery, sliced

1 seeded cucumber, sliced

2 cups mixed sprouts (e.g. mung bean, soy bean and alfalfa)

1 cup mixed salad herbs of your choice (e.g. parsley, chives, basil, dill, cilantro etc.)

Combine all the ingredients and toss with one of our salad dressings. Serve on shredded lettuce.

Green Beans in Ginger Salad

Serves 4

1½ inch (3.75cm) piece ginger root, peeled and finely grated

1 tsp ground fennel seeds (optional) or 2 tbsp finely cut fresh fennel leaves

1 lb (450g) green beans, trimmed and sliced diagonally

2 heaped tbsp finely chopped fresh mint

2 heaped tbsp finely chopped fresh chives

1 tsp cold-pressed virgin olive oil

Place 2 cups water into a saucepan, add the ginger and fennel and cook for 2-3 minutes. Add the beans, mint and chives and stir gently. Cook until the beans are just tender. Drain and refrigerate. Toss in oil before serving.

Avocado Salad with Walnuts
Serves 4 - 6
1 red butter lettuce
3 avocados, peeled and sliced
½ red onion finely sliced
1 lemon juiced
4 tablespoons cold pressed olive oil
½ cup walnuts chopped
salt and pepper to taste

Wash and dry the lettuce and place into a bowl. Add avocados, lemon juice and oil, fold nuts and onion through salad and toss well.

Walnut, Celery and Fennel Salad
Serves 4
1 fennel bulb, washed and chopped
3 sticks celery with some leaves on, washed and finely chopped
1.8 oz (50g) walnuts, shelled and roughly chopped

Pour over special dressing below to serve

Special fruity oil dressing:
1 tbsp sesame oil
2 tbsp olive oil
1 tsp mayonnaise
1 tsp grainy mustard
juice of 1 lemon or 1 tbsp white wine vinegar
1 tbsp apple juice
freshly ground black pepper

Blend all ingredients together until smooth.

Bamboo Shoots, Carrot and Raisin Salad

Serves 4
1 cup bamboo shoots (fresh or canned)
1 cup raw carrot, grated
1 cup finely sliced radish
1 cup diced scallions / green onions
½ cup raisins
1 heaped tbsp finely grated orange zest

Combine all the ingredients and toss with one of our salad dressings.

Oriental Salad

Serves 6
4 oz (110g) snow peas, topped and tailed
½ Chinese cabbage, finely shredded
8 oz (225g) mung bean sprouts
14 oz (400g) canned whole baby corn spears, drained
4 oz (110g) fresh button mushrooms, thinly sliced
1 red bell pepper (capsicum), cut into long thin slices
8 scallions / green onions, julienned, retaining green parts

Steam snow peas for 2 minutes and plunge into cold water (about 30 seconds). Drain then combine with all the other ingredients and the special dressing.

Special dressing:
2 tbsp cold-pressed virgin olive oil
1 tbsp vinegar (white-wine, balsamic, or apple cider)
Juice of ½ lemon freshly squeezed
1 tbsp soy sauce
1 garlic clove, minced (optional)
1 heaped tbsp almond slivers
2 heaped tbsp toasted sesame seeds

Mix all the ingredients together and pour over the Oriental salad. Toss and serve.

Seafood Salad

Serves 4

1 lb (450g) sea scallops
1 lb (450g) cooked peeled shrimp (prawns)
4oz (110g) snow peas
3 stalks celery, finely chopped
1 red bell pepper (capsicum), julienned
6 scallions / green onions
14 oz (400g) can water chestnuts, drained and sliced

Poach scallops in boiling water for 2 minutes and remove with a slotted spoon, set aside to cool. Steam snow peas for 2 minutes then plunge into iced water for 30-40 seconds to stop overcooking. Drain snow peas. Mix all the ingredients in a bowl and toss with special dressing.

Special dressing:

1 garlic clove, minced
4 tbsp vinegar (apple cider, balsamic, or white-wine)
2 tbsp cold-pressed virgin olive oil
1 tbsp cold-pressed sesame oil
1 tbsp dry mustard powder (do not use if you don't like it spicy!)
4 tbsp soy sauce
1 pinch chilli powder (if desired)

Combine all ingredients for the dressing in a screw top jar and shake vigorously.

Mixed Bean Salad

Serves 4

½ cup dried chickpeas
½ cup dried red kidney beans
½ cup dried butter beans
½ cup dried black-eyed beans

Soak all the beans for 12 hours, then wash and drain.
Fill a saucepan with cold fresh water, add the beans and bring very slowly to a boil (takes about 30 minutes). Simmer over a low heat for 40 minutes until tender. Rinse, drain and refrigerate while preparing the special dressing.

Special dressing:

¼ cup cold-pressed virgin olive oil
2 tbsp lemon juice, freshly squeezed
1 garlic clove, minced
3 scallions / green onions, finely chopped
1 tsp dry mustard
Fresh parsley, finely chopped
Fresh cilantro (coriander), finely chopped

Mix the first five ingredients well, then pour over cold beans and toss. Sprinkle with parsley and coriander before serving.
This salad is nice with grilled fish.
One of our other dressings may be used if preferred.

Cherry Tomato, Avocado and Grapefruit Salad

Serves 2 - 4

1 radicchio lettuce
1 medium avocado, peeled and diced
1 grapefruit, peeled and divided into small segments
2 cups cherry tomatoes
¼ cup chopped chives

Place the lettuce leaves on plate. Arrange avocado, grapefruit and tomatoes on top. Choose one of our delicious salad dressings, drizzle it all over. Garnish with chives and serve.

Mushrooms with Walnuts and Walnut Oil Dressing
Serves 4

8 oz (225g) small button mushrooms (champignons)
7 tbsp vinegar (apple cider, balsamic or white-wine)
2 tbsp cold pressed walnut oil
2 tsp Dijon mustard
Freshly ground black pepper and sea salt to taste
1 tsp of date and apple chutney, or chutney of choice
5 tbsp finely chopped walnuts

Clean the mushrooms and remove stalks and slice finely. Mix together the vinegar, oil, mustard, pepper, salt and chutney. Add walnuts and chill. Coat the mushrooms with dressing just prior to serving

Garden Fresh Green Salad
Serves 4

½ lettuce washed and torn
10 small spinach leaves, washed and torn
½ romaine lettuce, washed and torn
½ cup snow pea sprouts
1 cup finely chopped watercress
½ cup finely chopped fresh dill
1 red onion, finely chopped
1 garlic clove, minced (optional)
4 tbsp fresh cilantro (coriander), chopped
Juice of 1 lime, freshly squeezed
2 heaped tbsp parsley, chopped

Combine all ingredients and serve with one of our lovely dressings.

Avocado, Mango and Lime Salad

Serves 2 - 4

2 red butter lettuces, washed and torn
1 avocado, peeled and chopped
1 fresh mango, peeled and diced
1 small green bell pepper (capsicum), finely chopped
1 small red bell pepper (capsicum), finely chopped
6 scallions / green onions, finely chopped
1 heaped tbsp fresh parsley, finely chopped
1 heaped tbsp fresh chives, finely chopped

Arrange the lettuce leaves on a platter. Combine all other ingredients and mix together with the special dressing. Place on top of lettuce.

Special dressing:

¼ cup cold pressed olive oil or avocado oil
¼ cup freshly squeezed lime juice
1 garlic clove, minced (optional)
1 heaped tbsp dried tarragon
1 heaped tbsp finely chopped fresh cilantro (coriander)
Freshly ground black pepper and sea salt to taste

Combine all ingredients and mix well.

Beansprout Salad

Serves 2 - 4

2 oz (50g) sprouted soy beans
2 apples, grated
6 oz (175g) sprouts of choice such as alfalfa, mung bean, mustard seed etc.
4 oz (100g) canned sweet corn, or cooked & sliced off cob
4 oz (100g) red bell pepper (capsicum), seeded & chopped
4 scallions / green onions

Toss all ingredients together and drizzle over one of our salad dressings.

Cruciferous Vegetable Salad with Herb Vinegar
This salad is high in sulphur to support liver detoxification and cleansing
Serves 4 - 6
½ cauliflower, broken into florets
3 cups broccoli florets
3 slices lemon
¼ cup each finely chopped mint and parsley
2 cups herb or tarragon vinegar

Lightly cook the cauliflower and broccoli in boiling water with slices of lemon. Drain. Remove the lemon then plunge vegetables into icy water for 30-40 seconds to prevent overcooking. Drain well. Sprinkle with mint and parsley and toss in herb vinegar.
Chill for 2-4 hours and toss again. Drain and serve. Alternatively, any of our other dressings may be used if you prefer them to herb vinegar.

Crustacean Salad
Any cooked seafood, such as crayfish, shrimps (prawns), crab-meat, lobster or a mixture of these, may be used in this recipe.
Serves 2 - 4
1 heaped tsp Madras curry powder
2 tbsp Mayonnaise (page 103)
1 mango, peeled and mashed
1 heaped tbsp finely chopped chives
1 heaped tbsp finely chopped fresh dill
2.2 lb (1 kg) fresh cooked seafood
1 lettuce, washed and crisped in refrigerator

Stir the curry powder into mayonnaise. If the mixture is too thick add 1 tbsp milk. Add mashed mango, chives and dill and stir well. Shell seafood. Make boats from lettuce leaves. Top with the seafood and mango mayonnaise.

Fetta Cheese, Pea and Mint Salad

Serves 4

7 oz (200g) Greek style fetta cheese
1 cup fresh peas or use frozen peas
7 oz (200g) snow peas, trimmed
5 oz (150g) sugar snap peas, trimmed
2 tbsp fresh mint leaves, finely chopped
1 tbsp white wine vinegar
¼ cup olive oil

Boil water in saucepan. Place peas in boiling water for 2 minutes then add sugar snap peas and snow peas and boil for 1 minute - drain. Plunge in a large bowl chilled water for 2 minutes - drain and pat dry with paper towel.

Sprinkle mint onto a plate and roll fetta in mint to coat. Cut fetta into bite sized cubes.

Add fetta, oil and vinegar to peas and gently mix through. This is nice served with lamb loin chops.

Asparagus and Lettuce Salad

Serves 6

1 butter lettuce, washed and crisped in refrigerator
1 red leaf lettuce, washed and crisped in refrigerator
1 red butter lettuce, washed and crisped in refrigerator
3 bunches fresh asparagus
1 red onion, finely sliced
4 tbsp parmesan or mature cheddar cheese grated

Wash and dry all lettuce leaves then tear into bite-sized pieces removing stalks. Chop the base off asparagus and steam on high for 3 minutes. Then plunge asparagus into icy water for 30 - 40 seconds, then drain well.

Cut asparagus into bite-sized pieces. Combine all ingredients and toss with oil and vinegar dressing. Sprinkle cheese on top. (French dressing is nice with this salad).

Apple, Carrot and Beet Salad

Serves 4

1 large Granny Smith apple
2 carrots
1 medium beet
Juice of 1 lime
2 tbsp cold-pressed olive oil
Pinch sea salt
Freshly ground black pepper
½ tsp honey
1 red butter lettuce
1 butter lettuce

Grate the apple, carrots and beet. Place the lime juice, oil, salt, pepper, and honey into a screw-top jar and shake. Arrange washed and dried lettuce leaves on plates. Place some of the grated mixture into the center of each leaf. Spoon the dressing over the top.

Coleslaw

Serves 4

1 cup grated carrot
3 cups shredded cabbage (center stalks removed)
1 cup diced green apple
½ cup raw walnuts, chopped
½ cup sunflower seeds
½ cup raisins
½ cup finely sliced red bell pepper (capsicum)

Toss all ingredients with one of our lovely dressings. It is nice with Mayonnaise (page 103).

Arugula and Apple Salad

Serves 4

1 sweet apple
3 large handfuls fresh arugula
1 small red onion
1 cup parmesan cheese roughly grated
½ cup pine nuts dry roasted

Dressing:

salt and pepper
¼ cup unsweetened apple juice or apple cider
¼ cup cold pressed olive oil
¼ tsp mustard
1 tsp honey

To make dressing:

Whisk all ingredients together in a bowl and add some freshly grated nutmeg to taste. Whisk together again. Wash and chop arugula, pat dry. Add arugula to bowl. Peel apple and slice thinly and cut into halves and add apple to bowl. Chop onion very finely and add onion to bowl. Dry roast pine nuts on low heat in fry pan, watch closely so not to burn - put nuts aside for serving. Add dressing, parmesan cheese and pine nuts to salad. Toss and serve.

Courgette Salad

Serves 4 - 6

8 small courgettes (zucchini)
1 cup chopped basil
1 red onion, finely chopped
1 green bell pepper (capsicum), finely sliced
1 red bell pepper (capsicum), finely sliced

Cut courgettes into 2 inch (5 cm) slices and steam over boiling water until just tender. Drain and place in a serving dish. Toss with other ingredients and a dressing of your choice.

Pickled Beets
Serves 4
1 bunch beets
1 medium red onion
1 large bay leaf
½ cup organic apple cider vinegar
1 tbsp honey
1 clove
black pepper and salt
juice ¼ lemon
½ tsp fresh mustard or approx 20 mustard seeds

Wash and peel beet and chop into chunky pieces. Fill saucepan with water, add beet and spices (water should cover the beet generously). Heat, then add honey. Cook on low heat for around 45 mins, add chopped red onion and cook on low heat for another 25 mins, covered. Check occasionally so not to overcook. This dish can be eaten hot as a side dish or used to make the beet salad.

Beet Salad
Serves 4
10 pieces homemade beets (from previous recipe)
1 handful fresh young beet leaves or arugula, washed and chopped
1 small red onion
1 celery stick with leaves finely chopped
½ bunch fresh basil, chopped finely
10 walnuts or ½ cup pine nuts
9 oz (250g) goat cheese or fetta cheese, in bite sized pieces

Dressing:
cold pressed olive oil
apple cider vinegar
½ tsp mustard
1 tsp honey

Chop all herbs and onion and place in bowl. Dry roast walnuts/pine nuts in a skillet or fry pan on low heat, watch carefully not to burn. Put nuts aside to serve. Just before serving, add the beet and goat cheese to salad bowl.

Whisk olive oil, honey, apple cider vinegar and mustard in a bowl and pour over salad and add nuts on top and serve.

Chickpea Salad

Serves 4 - 6

2 x 14 oz (400g) cans organic chickpeas, washed & drained
1 large red onion, finely chopped
1 large corn cob or 2 medium sized cobs
1 small red bell pepper (capsicum), cored, seeded, thinly sliced
1 bunch fresh cilantro (coriander), washed and finely chopped
2 celery sticks with leaves finely chopped
1 carrot, peeled and grated

Pre-cook corn cob and allow to cool. Cut kernels from cob and set aside.

Toss together all salad ingredients in a large bowl and drizzle salad dressing over salad and serve immediately.

Dressing:

½ orange, juiced
1 tsp ginger, finely grated
½ cup cold pressed olive oil
½ lemon, juiced
salt and pepper
1 tbsp cumin spice (not seeds)
pinch cayenne pepper
1 tbsp honey

Whisk ingredients together in a bowl and set aside.

Snow Pea and Avocado Salad

Serves 4

2 cups snow peas
1 red butter lettuce
1 large ripe avocado, peeled and diced
2 cups cherry tomatoes, halved
½ cup alfalfa sprouts
4 sprigs fresh basil, finely chopped

Top and tail the snow peas and steam for approximately 3 minutes until just tender, then plunge into icy water for 30 - 40 seconds to prevent overcooking. Drain.

Tear the washed and dried lettuce leaves into bite-sized pieces and arrange in the bottom of a salad bowl. Add avocado, tomatoes, snow peas, sprouts, and basil. Choose one of our lovely salad dressings and pour over salad.

Dips and spreads

Nut Cream

¾ cup fresh raw cashews
¾ cup almonds (blanched or with skins soaked off)
3 oranges, peeled and sectioned
1 apple, peeled and sectioned
1 tbsp natural honey or 2 pinches of stevia powder if a sweet taste is desired. Stevia is best for weight watchers.

If desired, add some vanilla extract and/or ground nutmeg and cinnamon. Grind nuts and add to the fruit. Place this mixture in a blender and blend until fine and creamy.

This is nice on top of fresh fruit salad or with some cheese.

Tofu and Salmon Spread

7 oz (210g) canned salmon, water-packed
3½ oz (100g) tofu
2 scallions / green onions, finely chopped
1 heaped tbsp finely chopped fresh cilantro (coriander)
2 sprigs fresh mint, finely chopped
Juice of ½ lemon
Freshly ground black pepper

Combine all ingredients, mash to a paste and spread on Ryvita biscuits with cucumber and tomato.

Hummus

4 oz (125g) dried chickpeas
4 large garlic cloves, chopped
3 tbsp tahini
4 tablespoons sesame seeds
Juice of 3 lemons, freshly squeezed
1 teaspoon paprika

Soak the chickpeas overnight and discard skins. Drain.

Using fresh water, boil the soaked chickpeas for 1 hour and drain. Place the chickpeas in a blender and blend with the garlic until smooth. Set aside.

Place the sesame seeds in a grinder and grind until smooth. Add to chickpeas and garlic. Stir in the lemon juice, tahini and mix well. Sprinkle with paprika. Spread on Ryvita biscuits or have with sticks of carrot, courgettes (zucchini), celery, cucumber, snow peas and grated beet.

Note: If preferred, hummus can be bought ready-made at health food stores or supermarkets.

Salmon and Cheese Dip

14 oz (425g) can pink salmon, drained
juice of one lemon
¼ cup sour cream
2 gherkins, chopped
4 oz (120g) mayonnaise (sugar free)
9 oz (250g) cottage or ricotta cheese
1 tbsp chives, chopped
salt and pepper

In a blender place all ingredients and blend until smooth. Place in serving dish, cover and chill until required.

Avocado Dip

Mash 1 ripe avocado with freshly ground black pepper, sea salt, 2 finely chopped scallions / green onions, juice of ½ lemon and 2 tbsp olive oil.

Tahini and Yoghurt Dip

4 tbsp tahini
3 tbsp lemon juice
1 clove garlic, minced
pinch chilli powder
pinch sea salt
1 tsp hot chilli sauce (optional)
6 tbsp water
3 tbsp full fat plain acidophilus yoghurt

Combine tahini, lemon juice, garlic, salt, chilli powder, chilli sauce and mix well. As the mixture thickens add water and beat until sauce runs freely off spoon.
Add yoghurt and beat, mixture should be smooth and easy to pour.

Broad Bean Dip
18 oz (500g) broad beans, canned or dried
1 tsp cumin powder
1 tsp cardamom powder
2 cloves garlic crushed (optional)
½ lemon, freshly squeezed
½ cup cold pressed olive oil
1 whole chilli, seeded and diced (optional)

Cook beans in water with cumin, cardamom and garlic. Drain beans and retain juice. Add lemon juice, retrieve garlic and place with the beans. Puree all together with the oil – add more juice if needed.

Breakfast Recipes

Quick Berry High Protein Milk Shake
1 cup any milk (unsweetened and sugar free)
3 tbsp canned full cream coconut milk
1 ½ cup crushed ice or ½ cup water
1 cup berries – fresh or frozen
2 - 3 tbsp Synd-X Slimming Protein Powder

Blend together and serve immediately.

Strawberries, raspberries, blackberries, blueberries or mixed berries can be used in this shake. Berries contain organic acids that help to lower insulin and are a slimming fruit to choose.

Passionfruit is also nice in this smoothie.

LSA

LSA stands for Linseeds, Sunflower seeds and Almonds and this mixture proved to be very popular in The Liver Cleansing Diet Book.

To make your own LSA, use:
3 cups whole linseeds (flaxseeds)
2 cups whole sunflower seeds
1 cup whole almonds

Mix and grind together until a fine powder. A regular coffee grinder or a food processor will do the job nicely.
Store LSA in a dark colored glass jar (must be air tight) in the refrigerator or pack into sealed plastic bag and store in freezer.
LSA mixture has a slightly sweet and nutty taste and can be added to smoothies and yoghurt, sprinkled on fruit, vegetables, or just about anything. It is a good source of protein, essential fatty acids, minerals, and fiber and low in carbohydrates. LSA is also good to prevent constipation.

Low Carb High Fiber Muesli

Serves 4 - 6
2 cups rolled oats
½ cup seedless raisins
1 cup rye flakes or rice bran
½ cup sunflower seeds
½ cup chopped dried apples
¼ teaspoon ground nutmeg
½ cup shelled walnuts
¼ teaspoon ground cinnamon
½ cup almonds
¼ cup pepita seeds

Combine and mix all ingredients in a large bowl. Place in an airtight container and refrigerate.
Fresh fruit, such as strawberries, prunes, kiwifruit, oranges,

apples, or any fruit of your choice may be added along with LSA to your cereal. Serve with milk, diluted coconut milk, unsweetened soy milk, or with plain acidophilus yoghurt.

Note: if you have irritable bowel syndrome you may grind the seeds and nuts into a fine powder before adding them to the other ingredients.

No Grain High Protein Low Carb Cereal

Equal parts of –
Psyllium husks
Whey protein powder or Synd-X Slimming Protein Powder
Linseeds (flaxseeds)
Pumpkin seeds
Sunflower seeds
Almonds
Cashew nuts - chopped

Grind linseeds, pumpkin seeds, sunflower seeds and almonds in a food processor. Mix all ingredients together.
Serve this cereal with milk (dairy, unsweetened soy milk or coconut milk) or 3 tbsp of plain acidophilus yoghurt. When using coconut milk on a cereal it is best to dilute it with water – use 4 tbsp full cream canned coconut milk to one cup water, or use more water if it tastes too thick. One piece fresh fruit may be added if desired.
Note: this grain free, gluten free home made cereal is very low in carbs and is excellent for constipation or irritable bowel syndrome. It also helps to lower cholesterol levels.

Scrambled Tofu

Serves 3
2 tablespoons water
1 ½ lb (680g) tofu chopped
2 small onions, peeled and diced

1 tbsp minced garlic
½ green bell pepper (capsicum), finely chopped
½ cup fresh mushrooms, sliced
4 tbsp cold-pressed virgin olive oil
½ tbsp brown mustard
2 tbsp miso or soy sauce
1 tsp curry powder
4 tbsp finely chopped fresh mint or parsley
¼ tsp chilli powder
¼ tsp freshly ground black pepper
¼ tsp sea salt

Heat the water in a skillet or wok, add the tofu, onions, garlic, bell pepper and mushrooms, then add the oil. Cook for 8 - 10 minutes over a medium heat.

Mix the mustard and miso together in a bowl and pour over the tofu mixture in the wok. Stir in the curry powder, mint, chilli powder, black pepper, and salt and continue cooking for 6 - 8 minutes until most of the liquid in the wok evaporates. Serve hot with a salad or cooked vegetables.

You may sprinkle with LSA to increase the protein content.

Eggs - Healthy ways to cook them
(use free range or organic eggs)

Curried Eggs: Boil 4 eggs for 10 minutes, mash with 2 tablespoons unsweetened milk and 1 tablespoon curry powder and mix well.

Perfect Poached Eggs: Fill a nonstick pan with water, add 1 tablespoon apple cider vinegar and bring to a boil. Add eggs and reduce heat to cook to desired consistency. Make sure there is enough water to cover the eggs.

Hard Boiled or **Soft Boiled Eggs** are also healthy.

Avoid frying eggs at high temperatures, as their cholesterol turns to unhealthy oxidized 'oxy-cholesterol'.

Main Meal Recipes

Frittata

Serves 3 - 4
4 large eggs
3 tbsp flat leafed parsley, chopped
7 oz (95g) can salmon, drained (optional)
1 cup basil, chopped
1 leek, washed well and cut thinly
2 tsp olive oil
2 carrots, peeled and grated
1 clove garlic, crushed
2 oz (60g) butter
2 tbsp cheddar or parmesan cheese, grated (optional)
salt and black pepper

Melt butter, add leek and garlic and cook for 3 minutes (avoid browning). Add carrot and place lid on pan and cook for 10 minutes on low heat - allow to cool. Beat the eggs enough to combine them. Heat olive oil in suitable pan and arrange salmon on bottom, then arrange carrot, leek and basil on top of salmon. Pour in the egg mixture to cover base of pan - lift edges of frittata with a spatula so uncooked egg mixture runs underneath.

When frittata sets on top, turn it over. Serve hot with parsley and grated cheese sprinkled on top. Delicious served with a fresh garden salad.

Omelette

Serves 1
3 eggs
1 oz (30g) butter
1 tbsp milk
salt and pepper

Beat eggs in a bowl until yolks and whites are combined. Stir in milk, salt and pepper. Heat butter until it covers the base of a pan and pour beaten eggs into pan. Over moderate heat, draw outer edges of mixture into the center of pan with a spatula until eggs are lightly set. Tilt pan away from you to enable easy rolling or folding of omelette. Tip omelette onto warmed plate.

For variety, fillings can be added inside folded omelette – suggestions include grated cheese, cooked asparagus, seafood or mushrooms, salmon, goat or fetta cheese and fresh herbs.

Crispy Asian Green Vegetables
Great served with grilled fish or canned fish on the side
Serves 2 - 3
1 cup Chinese cabbage, shredded – if unavailable use regular cabbage
2 bunches baby bok choy
1 bunch Chinese broccoli – if unavailable use regular broccoli
2 tbsp cold pressed sesame oil or olive oil
2 tbsp oyster sauce
Juice of one small lemon
1 tbsp sesame seeds
Freshly ground black pepper
½ tsp sea salt

Soak all vegetables in cold water for 30 mins, then rinse. Trim off dead or damaged parts/leaves. Cut bok choy in half lengthwise. Cut off hard end of Chinese broccoli and chop into pieces. Boil water in a saucepan with the sea salt. Cook all vegetables in the boiling water for 2 - 3 mins, then drain. Heat oil in a wok on medium heat, add oyster sauce and lemon juice, stir, then add vegetables and cook for 2 mins on low heat. Serve sprinkled with sesame seeds.

Grilled Tomatoes

Halve the tomatoes, then make small slits in each tomato half and place a sliver of garlic in each. Lightly brush with cold-pressed virgin olive oil, sprinkle with pepper and salt and grill.

Cooked Mushrooms

Use as many finely sliced button or field mushrooms as desired.

Heat a nonstick pan which has been brushed on the base and sides with cold-pressed virgin olive oil. Add mushrooms, then soy sauce and milk. Cook on a low heat.

Aubergine and Cilantro Salad

Serves 4

2 small aubergine (eggplants), halved lengthways
2 tbsp olive oil
½ cup fresh cilantro (coriander), chopped
1 tbsp orange juice
1 tbsp lemon juice
3 small courgettes (zucchini)

Cut aubergine into thin slices, place in a colander and lightly sprinkle with salt and stand for 15 minutes.

Cut courgettes lengthways into very thin slices (this is best done using a vegetable peeler) and set aside.

Wash aubergine and dry with paper towels.

Preheat grill, then brush both sides aubergine with oil and put on baking tray. Grill aubergine until lightly brown on both sides. Remove aubergine to cool.

In a salad bowl, place aubergine, courgettes, cilantro, juices, oil, salt and pepper and combine.

Stuffed Green Bell Peppers

Serves 4

17 oz (480g) mushrooms thinly sliced
8 medium green bell peppers (capsicums)
3 tbsp olive oil
5 scallions / green onions, thinly sliced
1 cup fresh basil, chopped
7 oz (200g) parmesan cheese or cheddar cheese, grated
6 oz (170g) cooked green lentils
salt and pepper
3 oz (80ml) hot water
1 vegetable stock cube
4 ripe tomatoes, chopped
1 tbsp fresh rosemary chopped or 1 tsp dried rosemary
2 cloves garlic, peeled and crushed
16 oz (450g) lean veal or lamb, ground
8½ oz (250g) celery, thinly sliced

Cut tops off bell peppers, core, seed and rinse well then soak peppers in hot water for 4 minutes. Drain and pat dry with paper towels.

Preheat the oven to 375°F (190°C).

In a large pan heat olive oil. Place onions, mushrooms, celery in pan and cook for 3 minutes on low heat. Add meat, garlic and cook on medium heat until meat is brown. Add stock cube, hot water, rosemary, tomatoes, salt, pepper and simmer for 8 minutes. Add cooked lentils and chopped basil to mixture, stir well.

Fill each pepper two-thirds with mixture and sprinkle with half of parmesan cheese. Top with remaining mixture and sprinkle with rest of parmesan cheese.

Place stuffed peppers in baking dish and bake for around 15 minutes.

Roast vegetables

Great with meat or salad - veggies never tasted so good!

Serves 4

2 parsnips

1 leek

3 carrots

1 large turnip

1 large sweet potato

1 brown onion

2 sprigs fresh rosemary, chopped finely from the stalk

2 bay leaves

2 tbsp cold pressed olive oil

Sea salt and black pepper

1 tsp thyme

1 tsp mixed spice

1 tbsp Old Bay Spice or equivalent

1 tbsp tamari

Cut all vegetables into thick strips like large potato wedges, except onion and leek. Slice onion into medium slices and cut leek into large pieces.

In a large baking dish put oil and tamari. Roll vegetables into this mixture coating well. Add all the spices. Bake in a moderate oven for 30 minutes in a covered pan. Remove from oven, stir and place back in oven, uncovered for 20 to 30 minutes to brown.

Tip - how to make your own version of Old Bay Spice

Combine 2 ½ tbsp paprika, 2 tbsp sea salt, 2 tbsp garlic powder, 1 tbsp black pepper, 1 tbsp onion powder, 1 tbsp cayenne pepper, 1 tbsp dried leaf oregano and 1 tbsp dried thyme.

Mashed Spicy Sweet Potatoes

Serves 4

3 large sweet potatoes or yams
1 tbsp Old Bay Spice or equivalent
salt and pepper
1 tbsp butter
½ cup milk
freshly grated whole nutmeg to taste

Wash, peel and chop potatoes. Place in steamer and cook until very soft. In a mixing bowl place hot potatoes, butter, milk and all spices. Mash with a masher or fork until smooth. Adjust spice to taste - serve hot.

Colcannon potato dish

Serves 4

1 tbsp chopped chives
4 oz (110g) green cabbage, shredded finely
4 oz (110g) red cabbage, shredded finely
5 tbsp milk
8 oz (225g) sweet potatoes diced
2 scallions / green onions, chopped
1 tsp nutmeg, freshly grated
1 tbsp butter, melted
½ organic vegetable stock cube
½ cup water

Steam cabbage in steamer until tender. In another saucepan heat milk, water and stock cube and add diced potatoes and onion. Cook covered on low heat until soft.
Add nutmeg and mash potato and onion mixture together.
Add cabbage and mix well.
Place mixture in heated Pyrex dish, make a small hole in center and add butter and serve immediately.

Quick Easy Chicken Stir Fry

(chicken can be replaced with seafood or tofu)

Serves 4

8 oz (225g) chicken fillet, boned and skinned

1 tsp sesame oil

2 – 3 tbsp olive oil

2 tbsp oyster sauce

1 tbsp rice vinegar

1 tsp lemon grass, finely chopped

1 tsp fresh ginger root, chopped

½ tsp garlic minced

2 tsp fish sauce

4 small red chillies (optional)

2 oz (55g) snow peas

1 small bell pepper (capsicum), cored and cubed

2 oz (55g) can bamboo shoots, sliced and drained

1 tsp honey

salt pepper

Cut chicken, seafood or tofu into bite sized cubes and place in bowl with fish sauce, salt and pepper. Leave to marinate for 30 minutes.

Heat olive oil in frying pan or wok, add ginger, chillies, lemon grass and garlic and stir fry for 30 seconds. Add chicken pieces (or seafood or tofu) and stir fry several minutes. Add vegetables and cook for 2 to 3 minutes whilst stirring. Add honey, oyster sauce, vinegar and 3 tbsp water (or chicken stock). Stir well to blend, bring to a boil and add sesame oil.

Serve hot with flat rice noodles or wild rice.

Spicy Chicken Portuguese Style

Serves 4

50 oz (1.4kg) whole chicken
2 cups baby arugula, washed and chopped
lemon wedges to serve

Spicy marinade:

1 tbsp cold pressed olive oil
½ cup fresh oregano leaves, chopped
1/3 cup freshly squeezed lemon juice
2 small red chillies, finely chopped
1 long green chilli, finely chopped
2 tsp finely grated lemon rind
1 ½ tsp paprika
4 garlic cloves, crushed

Make the marinade by combining in a bowl the oregano, garlic, oil, lemon rind, lemon juice, chilli and paprika.

Rinse chicken thoroughly inside and out with cold running water and dry with paper towels. Place chicken, breast side down, on a chopping board. With scissors cut along each side of backbone and discard backbone. Turn chicken over and press on breast bone until it breaks.

Place chicken in baking dish. Rub both sides of chicken with marinade and cover. Refrigerate for 3 to 4 hours.

Preheat barbecue, char grill on high with hood closed. Cook chicken, skin side down for 20 minutes or until brown and crispy. Reduce heat to medium. Continue cooking for 45 minutes, turning occasionally until brown and cooked through.

Serve chicken with arugula and lemon wedges.

You may replace the chicken with fish, shellfish, turkey or pork as they all suit this marinade.

Lamb Curry - North Indian Style

Serves 4

18 oz (500g) fresh lean lamb forequarter, diced
2 tsp cold pressed olive oil
1 large onion, sliced
1 tsp ginger root, freshly grated
3 cloves garlic, crushed
½ tsp chilli powder (optional)
½ cup canned coconut milk
½ cup chicken stock or ½ organic vegetable stock cube
1 tsp of each – ground cardamom, garam masala, cumin,
½ bunch fresh cilantro (coriander)

Preheat oven to 350°F (180°C). Heat oil in a large heavy based casserole dish, add onions and fry for 3 mins, add ginger and garlic cook for 1 min then add spices and cook 1 min. Add lamb, cook for 4 mins, reduce heat to low, add coconut milk, cilantro and stock. Cover casserole dish, cook in oven for 2 to 2½ hours, stirring occasionally until meat is tender. Serve with a fresh green and tomato salad.

Chicken and Egg Salad

Serves 4

4 boneless chicken breasts
6 hard boiled eggs, cut into slices
30 black olives, stones removed
1 tsp sweet paprika
1 small lettuce, washed, shredded and chopped
5 sticks celery, chopped into fine slices
1 carrot, shredded
3.5 oz (100g) vintage cheese, crumbled
salt and pepper

Grill chicken breasts until tender, allow to cool and cut into thin slices. Sprinkle eggs with paprika then mix with all ingredients. Serve with dressing of vinegar and olive oil.

Veal with Cashew Nuts
Serves 4

18 oz (500g) fresh veal (organically raised on grass is ideal)
2 tsp cold pressed olive oil
1 tbsp soy sauce
2 cloves garlic, crushed
¼ cup fresh unsalted raw cashew nuts
1 bell pepper (capsicum), thinly sliced
1 carrot, cut into strips
2 broccoli florets, washed and chopped
1 cup snow peas, washed and trimmed
1 leek, washed and chopped finely
2 tsp ginger root, freshly grated

Slice meat thinly. Heat oil in wok and stir fry ginger and garlic for 1 min. Add veal strips and stir fry for 4 mins. Add all the vegetables, stir in soy sauce and cook until tender. Add cashews, and heat for 1 min. Serve with side salad.

Lemon and Herb Grilled Snapper
Serves 4

4 x 18 oz (500g) each whole baby snapper, cleaned
½ cup freshly squeezed lemon juice
½ inch (1 cm) fresh ginger, peeled and thinly sliced
1 lemon, sliced into 4 wedges to serve
1 lemon, halved lengthways thinly sliced
2 tbsp fresh dill chopped, reserving 4 stems
1 tbsp fresh cilantro (coriander), chopped
3 scallions / green onions, thinly sliced
olive oil

Wash fish inside and out with cold running water, then dry fish with paper towel. Make 3 cuts, ½ inch (1cm) deep into fleshy part on each side of fish. Preheat barbecue on high with hood closed. Take 4 pieces of foil and brush

inside of foil pieces with olive oil. Drizzle over each fish 1 tbsp lemon juice and 1½ tsp olive oil, then sprinkle with ¼ chopped dill, ½ chopped cilantro, ginger slices and salt and pepper. Place lemon slices, rest of dill and cilantro into fish cavities. Fold up the foil to enclose fish into parcels. Reduce barbecue heat to medium and place fish parcels on barbecue plate. Cook covered for 15 mins and to check if cooked, use a small knife to gently separate flesh at thickest part; if flesh is white up to the bone, it is done. Open parcels and using spatula place fish on warmed plates. Drizzle with small amount of olive oil, top with onion.
Serve with lemon wedges and fresh garden salad.

Baked Cod Fish

Serves 4
4 cod fillets, skinned
2 tsp fresh basil, chopped
2 tomatoes, peeled and diced
1 green bell pepper (capsicum), diced
1 clove garlic, crushed
1 onion, finely chopped
½ lemon or lime, juiced
3 tbsp olive oil
salt and pepper
lemon slices to garnish

Brush 4 large squares of foil with oil and preheat oven to 375°F (190°C).
Mix together the garlic, basil, tomatoes, bell pepper, onion. Place one cod fillet on each piece of foil and place mixture on top of each fillet. Drizzle with remaining oil and lemon juice. Sprinkle with salt and pepper. Fold the foil to make the four parcels. Place parcels on a baking sheet. Bake for 20 - 30 mins.
Unwrap parcels and place fish and vegetables and juices on warmed plates to serve. Garnish with lemon slices.

Grilled Prawns

Serves 4

1 lb (450g) large (king) prawns
2 tbsp tomato paste
1 clove garlic, crushed
6 tbsp olive oil
1 lemon, juiced
1 tbsp fresh basil, chopped
cayenne pepper, salt and ground black pepper

Remove heads and legs from prawns and rinse. Cut into halves lengthwise but leave end of tail in one piece so prawn looks like a butterfly. Place prawns in a bowl and pour over half the lemon juice and half the olive oil. Mix in garlic and leave for 30 minutes.

Preheat grill. Place prawns in a single layer on rack and place under hot grill for 4 minutes. The prawns should have curled (butterflied) and be pink.

In a side bowl mix together the remaining olive oil, lemon juice, tomato paste, basil, spices. This mixture can be served on the side to dip the prawns into. Serve prawns garnished with basil.

Teriyaki Fish Steaks

For the barbecue

Serves 4

4 x 7 oz (200g) fresh fish steaks – choose from tuna, snapper, salmon and/or barramundi
3 tsp soy or tamari sauce
2 cloves garlic, crushed
sea salt and black pepper

Wipe barbecue grill with paper towel soaked in olive oil.

Pre heat barbecue. Place fish steaks in shallow glass dish. Mix the tamari and garlic together and pour over fish and marinate for 40 minutes.

Place fish on hot barbecue grill and cook 4 to 5 minutes per side. Serve immediately with a fresh salad and/or roast vegetables.

Grilled Fish with a Spicy Flavor

Serves 4

1 ½ lb (700g) fish fillets – good choices are bream, snapper or mullet

2 cloves garlic, crushed

1 green chilli, finely chopped

1 tsp paprika

½ cup cilantro (coriander), leaves chopped

3 tbsp freshly squeezed lime juice

1 ½ tsp ground cumin seeds or cumin spice

3 tbsp olive oil

6 sprigs mint and lime wedges to serve

sea salt

Place fish fillets in a shallow ceramic dish. Mix all ingredients except mint and lime wedges and spoon mixture over fish. Cover and leave for 3 hours, turning every 30 minutes. Preheat the grill. Grill fish for 5 minutes on each side, basting with mixture occasionally.

Serve hot with mint and lime wedges with a garden salad.

Dessert Recipes

Stewed Fruits
This can be eaten hot or cold with plain full fat or low fat yoghurt or cream
Serves 2
1 large green apple
2 red apples
2 pears
2 nectarines
2 peaches

Spices
½ tsp freshly grated or powdered nutmeg
1 vanilla bean or 1 tsp vanilla essence
1 cinnamon stick or ½ tsp powdered cinnamon
2 cloves
½ tsp white stevia powder or more according to taste or you can use 2 tbsp of erythritol or xylitol or 1 tbsp honey

Peel the apples and pears. Core apples and de-stone other fruit. Cut fruit into bite sized pieces and put in saucepan on a low heat. Add all spices with 1 tbsp pure water or unsweetened apple juice. Cook on very low heat in covered saucepan for 30 minutes.
Serve alone or with plain acidophilus yoghurt or cream.

Stewed Fruit Crumble Pie
Use the stewed fruits recipe for the filling
Serves 2 - 4
Topping
2 cups No Grain Cereal (see recipe page 125) or Low Carb High Fiber Muesli (see recipe page 124)
½ cup crushed walnuts

½ tsp stevia powder or 2 tbsp xylitol or 1 tbsp honey
1 tbsp cold pressed olive oil
1 tsp cinnamon
1 tsp butter
1 tsp freshly grated nutmeg

Mix ingredients together in a bowl. Melt oil and butter and add to bowl. Place stewed fruit in Pyrex dish. Add the No Grain Muesli and spread evenly over the top of fruit. Grate a little extra nutmeg on top, then bake under griller until muesli turns golden.

Healthy Creamy Fruit Ice Cream

Serves 4
Use fruits of choice – such as any berries, banana, pears, rockmelon, etc.

2 cups fresh fruit, chopped
½ cup milk (unsweetened)
1 tsp honey
½ tsp stevia powder
1 tbsp agar agar (a natural equivalent to gelatine)
15 oz (425ml) can coconut cream
2 tbsp full fat plain yoghurt
3 tbsp cream

Mix all ingredients together in a food processor until smooth. Pour into container and freeze.
Serve in scoops with crushed almonds or with stewed fruit or poached pears.

Peachy Delights

Easy and quick to make!
Serves 4 - 6
30 oz (825g) peach halves
3½ oz (100g) plain acidophilus yoghurt
1 cup mixed dried fruit, chopped
1 tbsp orange juice
1 pinch ground cinnamon
½ cup toasted coconut

Arrange peach halves in individual serving dishes. Mix fruit juice with dried fruit and leave stand for ½ hour, then fold in yoghurt. Spoon mixture into the hollows of the peaches. Sprinkle with cinnamon and coconut.

Poached Pears

Serves 4
3 large pears, peeled and cored
½ cup dried apricots, chopped
½ cup shredded coconut
¼ cup almonds, chopped
1-2 sticks cinnamon
1 tsp honey or ½ tsp stevia powder
1 cup apple juice

Cut pears in half and lay center up in casserole dish. Mix together chopped apricots, coconut, almonds and cinnamon; add enough honey to bind mixture together. Divide the mixture evenly over the six pear halves. Add the apple juice slowly to the casserole.

Cover and bake in preheated oven at 350°F (180°C), approx 30 minutes.

Serve warm with our healthy ice cream.

CHAPTER FOURTEEN

Frequently asked liver questions

Can I eat dairy products if I have a fatty liver?

If you have a fatty liver I would recommend that the only dairy products you eat are –

- Plain (unflavored) yoghurt – this does not have to be reduced fat, although some people prefer this. Make sure that you avoid yoghurts that contain sugar or artificial sweetcners.

- Certain cheeses such as ricotta, pecorino, romano, vintage cheddar, fetta, cottage, ricotta and parmesan are suitable as they are high in protein and low in carbohydrates. You may have full fat or reduced fat cheeses but avoid processed sliced cheeses.

- Cows and goats milk are suitable and organic or biodynamic is best.

For some people with gallstones, dairy products can cause abdominal discomfort and bloating so they may tolerate only very small amounts.

You can use other milks such as unsweetened soymilk, rice milk, oat milk, almond milk, and canned coconut milk.

Coconut milk does not contain cholesterol but does contain saturated fat in the form of medium chain triglycerides. Coconut milk does not contain inflammatory proteins or hormones. For people with fatty liver coconut milk is not a problem provided it is diluted with water. For most patients with fatty liver, it's the carbohydrates in their diet that are the problem and provided the types of fat you are eating are unprocessed you will not find them a problem.

If you have a fatty liver you should dilute the canned coconut milk at least 50% with water.

Please check the labels on the milk containers as you must avoid milks with added sugar; if it tastes sweet it probably has sugar which will be turned into fat in your liver.

Some types of soymilk taste like a box of chemicals – have you ever found that? I personally do not like the taste of soymilk, but if you do, then it's ok to use it, but make sure it's free of genetically modified soybeans and don't buy brands with sugar added.

Are VERY High Protein Diets suitable for those with Fatty Liver?

In the long term, the answer is no, because they can increase the workload of the liver.

They may help you to lose weight temporarily and indeed quite quickly because they reduce insulin levels. For this reason we use them for a maximum of two weeks in some of our patients in our weight loss clinics.

In the long term very high-protein extremely low-carbohydrate diets are not suitable because they do not improve your liver function or heal damaged liver cells; thus despite all your hard work your liver will remain fatty. Indeed the high saturated fat content of some of the very well known "high protein diets" may increase your fatty liver problem and elevate LDL cholesterol levels, thus increasing your risk of cardiovascular disease. These things will reduce your life span so you may end up being the skinniest corpse in the cemetery!

Several popular high protein diets allow you to eat large amounts of cream, cream cheese, bacon, pork ribs, fried meats, fatty meats and preserved meats (such as ham, sausages, and pizza meats) and do not differentiate between the bad fats and the good fats.

Very high protein diets can cause a build up of the waste products of metabolism such as ammonia, urea and uric acid in your blood and this can over work the kidneys and liver. This is safe for a limited time of several weeks but only if you have normal liver and kidney function.

Some very high protein diets encourage the regular use of protein powders sweetened with the toxic artificial sweeteners called aspartame or aesculfame, which can cause problems with the liver and brain if large amounts are consumed.

Similarly diet sodas and soft drinks sweetened with aspartame or aesculfame will be toxic to your liver and brain if you consume them regularly. For more information visit www.dorway.com

Why don't very low-fat and very low-calorie diets work in Fatty Liver?

Because they lower the metabolic rate!

When you quit these extreme low calorie diets your metabolism is at an all time low; thus you will gain weight more rapidly than before you went on the diet.

These diets are too low in protein and healthy fats, and too high in carbohydrate, so that the blood insulin levels remain high, which keeps your hunger at excessive levels. You will never feel satisfied! Thus you cannot choose them as a way of life, as you will be hungry, tired and moody.

Many so called "diet foods" and "low fat foods" are highly processed to make them low in fat but they are very high in sugar and other hidden carbohydrates.

Check the labels of these low-fat diet foods and you may get a shock!

Their high sugar levels push up your insulin levels and remember insulin turns sugar into fat, especially in your liver. It's much healthier to eat full fat unflavored yoghurt than it is to eat the low fat "diet yoghurts," which are often high in sugar or artificial additives. You can add fresh fruit such as berries or passion fruit or Synd-X Slimming Protein Powder to plain unflavored yoghurt to make it sweeter.

Why do people with Fatty Liver often find it hard to start losing weight?

- Their liver has become accustomed to storing fat and it takes time to reverse this. A healthy liver is able to burn fat and pump excess fat out of the body through the bile. In those with a fatty liver, the reverse happens, so they just keep on getting fatter.

- The high levels of insulin make them very hungry. Indeed high insulin levels give you a ravenous appetite with cravings for carbohydrates.

Our program takes into account both of the above factors to enable you to escape from the vicious circle of ever increasing weight.

The menu plans and recipes in this book are not really a diet, but rather a "new way of eating", or more correctly "a very old way of eating", similar to the manner in which our ancient forebears ate before we distorted the food chain with high carbohydrate grains, refined sugar and hydrogenated vegetable oils.

Modern day processed foods have given us a convenient banquet of fatty liver promoting unnatural foods.

In contrast, the unprocessed natural low carbohydrate foods in my eating plan restore a healthy fat-burning metabolism.

It makes so much sense – just think about it for a minute! If you are battling with a fatty liver plus a ravenous hunger, your chances of long-term success are poor indeed.

My program gives you the two missing parts to the jigsaw puzzle –

- A healthy liver
- Normal insulin levels

Now you can see the big picture, and yes you can now understand why it has been so hard to achieve your goal. Your journey to a healthy weight is now going to become much easier, as by following my strategies you will be treating the causes of weight excess and poor health.

Can I drink alcohol if I have a fatty liver?

Many people enjoy a glass of wine or other alcohol on regular occasions to be social or to unwind and thus it is a common question for those who have a fatty liver – can I still drink alcohol?

Most people are aware that excess alcohol consumption over many years can cause serious liver disease and therefore ask about alcohol with reservation. They usually expect a resounding NO as the response.

However those of you that like the odd drink will be pleasantly surprised! Alcohol in moderation can be enjoyed when on a program to reverse fatty liver – BUT (well you knew there had to be one but!) there are important guidelines.

Alcohol as it is consumed is not what causes the damage to the liver – it is the substances known as metabolites that form during the breakdown of alcohol.

Ethanol (pure alcohol) is broken down in the liver to form acetaldehyde and damaging free radicals. So it is wise to allow time between alcohol intakes to allow the liver to fully metabolize and render safe the toxic metabolites of alcohol breakdown – for this reason it is recommended that you do not drink alcohol every day.

Alcohol consumption should be kept below 40 grams in a 24 hour period.

40 grams equals:

- 37 oz (1.1 liters) of beer
- 15 oz (0.44 liters) of wine
- 3.7 oz (0.11 liters) of spirits

Intakes above this have been associated with increased liver weight and increased incidence of fatty liver disease. Women are far more susceptible to alcohol-induced liver damage and therefore intake should be kept to no more than 20 – 30 grams of alcohol daily.

The best results were found in people that drank 1 to 3 days per week – so it is recommended to have days in between where no alcohol is consumed. This also gives the liver a chance to break down the metabolites of alcohol which, as stated, are the most harmful aspect of the alcohol consumption.

Types of alcohol

The best type of alcohol to choose in regards to weight control and insulin resistance is Spirits – such as gin, rum, vodka and whisky, as these have no carbohydrate content – however be very careful not to undo this benefit when choosing a drink mixer, as soft drinks including colas and lemonade, tonic water and other fizzy mixers can be very high in refined sugars. Better options are water, "on the rocks" (straight on ice) or soda water. If you miss the sweet taste of the mixer, you could try adding a little "Stevia" powder and citrus juice to the water or soda water.

Full strength beer and cider should be avoided or minimized, as 16oz or 1 pint (480ml) contains on average 17-18 grams of carbohydrate. Low carbohydrate beers are preferable. Avoid pre mixed drinks such as wine coolers and spritzers and sugary liqueurs as they are very high in sugar.

Carbohydrate Content of Alcohol

Alcohol Item *(serving size)*	Carbs *(g)*
Beer, regular (12 fl oz or 360mls)	13
Beer, light (12 fl oz or 360mls)	4.5
Wine, red (3½ oz or100mls)	1.75
Wine, rose (3½ oz or 100mls)	1.5
Wine, white (3½ oz or 100mls)	1
Cider, dry (16 fl oz or 480mls)	15
Gin, Rum, Vodka, Whisky (1 fl oz or 30mls)	0
Sherry (2 fl oz or 60mls)	3
Port (2 fl oz or 60mls)	6
Guinness (½ pint or 8 oz or 240mls)	4

Please Note: all carbohydrate values are approximate

Reference: Alcohol Clin Exp Res. 1993 Oct; 17(5):1112-7. Moderate Alcohol Consumption Has Beneficial Glycemic Effects Diabetes Care 2003; 26:1971-1978.

What is the role of liver tonics in fatty liver?

Liver Tonics

If you have a fatty liver a good liver tonic in powder or capsule form can improve your liver function. These liver tonics help to improve the liver's detoxification and fat burning functions and can stimulate repair of damaged liver cells. The liver is the most strategic organ in the body and therefore everyone, even the fit and healthy, need to take care of their liver in this chemical day and age.

Liver tonics are helpful for the following -

• An aid for weight reduction and fat burning

• An aid for those with high cholesterol and/or triglycerides

- Gall bladder dysfunction and gallstones
- Fluid retention and abdominal bloating
- Constipation (liver tonic powders are more effective than the capsules for a laxative effect)
- Irritable Bowel Syndrome
- Relief of digestive disorders
- Bad breath and coated tongue
- To rid the body of waste and promote elimination via a cleansing effect on the bowel
- Fatty liver induced by alcohol or poor diet
- Support for those people who are poor detoxifiers of drugs, or have multiple chemical or food allergies
- Syndrome X and diabetes
- Increased protection for people who work in high risk occupations such as:

  Painters, hairdressers, nail technicians, engineers, motor mechanics, agricultural workers, foundry workers, plumbers, electricians, plant and transport operators and some process and factory workers who are exposed to high loads of potential liver toxins such as petrochemicals, insecticides and solvents.

  Ensure that you use safe work practices, including gloves and masks, to protect your liver, if you are working around potential liver toxins.

  For more information on liver tonics, see page 41.

Adverse Reactions

If the patient is very toxic, the initial use of the full dose of a powerful liver tonic may cause excessive release of toxins resulting in headaches, nausea, abdominal cramps or diarrhea. Thus it is important to begin with a lower dose to avoid these unpleasant reactions. It is important to drink at least 10 glasses of pure water during the day.

How can I treat gall bladder problems naturally?

See www.liverdoctor.com/flb and click "Gall bladder" for indepth information. If you require specific help email us at fattyliver@liverdoctor.com

How long does it take to reverse a Fatty Liver?

This varies depending upon the degree of fatty liver that you have – more specifically the amount of inflammation and fat that exists in your liver.

If you have only a mild degree of fatty liver, this eating plan will work quickly. In other words you will start to lose weight within the first 2 weeks and the weight loss will be sustained.

If you have a very fatty liver the weight loss will be slower and you may have weight loss plateaus. A plateau is a flat line in weight loss when you find that weight loss stops for 2 to 3 weeks at a time. After the plateau your weight loss will resume provided you stick to the recommendations in this book.

It takes time to remove the excess fat from the liver and replace this fat with healthy metabolically active liver cells. It also takes time to reduce the inflammation in the liver and clear away the toxins that cause inflammation.

In some of my patients with advanced degrees of fatty liver it has taken up to 2 years to completely remove all the excess fat from the liver. Initial weight loss may be slow (say one pound or 0.5 kilogram per week), however the weight loss becomes sure and gradual and most importantly the weight will stay off permanently.

We are not just aiming for weight loss we are also aiming for a healthy liver free from damaging inflammation.

By renewing your liver we are helping you to have a healthy strong immune system that will protect you against many diseases.

The liver is the most important organ for longevity and good health. By removing the excess fat from the liver you will not only lose weight, but improve the metabolic imbalances of Syndrome X, such as high cholesterol and triglycerides, high uric acid and high insulin levels. This will result in cleaner blood vessels and a much lower risk of diabetes, heart disease and cancer. If you do not improve your liver function, long-term weight loss is not sustainable.

Do not become stressed or anxious by the fact that you have been diagnosed with a fatty liver, as it is able to be fully repaired, unlike many other organs in the body, which once damaged, remain permanently scarred and dysfunctional.

To see information on how doctors judge the degree of fatty liver in a patient, see www.liverdoctor.com/flb and click "Imaging".

Our Health Advisory Service in Phoenix Arizona receives many inspiring testimonials – to see some of these, visit www.liverdoctor.com/flb and click "Testimonials".

The Liverdoctor website also discusses a clinical study that we did on fatty liver reversal - see www.liverdoctor.com/flb and click "Clinical Study".

To obtain more help you may:

- Email us at fattyliver@liverdoctor.com or write to us at P.O. Box 5070, Glendale Phoenix AZ 85312
- Phone our FREE help line where you can speak to a naturopath on 1 623 334 3232
- Join our on-line weight loss club at www.weightcontroldoctor.com
- Get professional help by seeing a psychologist or food addiction counsellor.

  Wendy Perkins is a counselor who specializes in helping people who have addictions to food, drugs or alcohol - email her at change@scoastnet.com.au or visit her website www.couragetochange.com.au
- Visit www.confessionsofafatman.com

Blood tests for Liver Function

Some of the standard or routine blood tests that your doctor will order to check "liver function" are in reality only able to detect liver damage. These tests may not be sensitive enough to accurately reflect whether your liver is functioning at its optimum level. These tests will usually be abnormal in significant liver disease or liver distress; however, they can still give normal readings in some cases of mild liver disease. This is why imaging tests of the liver and gallbladder, such as ultrasound scans or CAT scans or MRI scans are important. These imaging tests can determine the degree of liver disease and if there are any tumors, cysts, gallstones or fatty accumulations, which change the texture of the liver.

Thankfully it is often possible to return abnormal liver function tests to normal with our dietary program and suitable liver tonics.

A routine blood test for liver function will be processed by an automated multi-channel analyzer, and will check the blood levels of the following:

- **Total Bilirubin**

    The normal range is:

    2 - 20 umol/L or 0.174 - 1.04 mg/dL. This test measures the amount of bile pigment in the blood.

    If blood levels of bilirubin become very elevated, the patient may have a yellow color to their skin and eyes and this is known as jaundice.

- **Liver Enzymes**

    AST *(aspartate aminotransferase)*, which was previously called SGOT, can also be elevated in heart and muscle diseases and is not liver specific.

    The normal range of AST is 0 - 45 U/L.

    ALT *(alanine aminotransferase)*, which was previously called SGPT, is more specific for liver damage.

    The normal range of ALT is 0 - 45 U/L.

ALP *(alkaline phosphatase)* is elevated in many types of liver disease, but also in non-liver related diseases.

The normal range of ALP is 30 - 120 U/L.

GGT *(gamma glutamyl transpeptidase)* is often elevated in those who use alcohol or other liver-toxic substances to excess.

The normal range of GGT is 0 - 45 U/L.

Why do all or some of these enzymes become elevated in cases of liver disease?

Normally these enzymes are mostly contained inside the liver cells; they only leak into the bloodstream when the liver cells are damaged. Thus, measuring liver enzymes is only able to detect liver damage and does not measure liver function in a highly sensitive way.

- **<u>Blood Proteins</u>**

These proteins are manufactured by the liver and are measured in the blood test for liver function.

Their normal ranges are as below:

Total protein: Normal range is 60 - 80g/L or 6 - 8g/dL

Serum albumin:

Normal range is 38 - 55g/L or 3.8 - 5.5g/dL

Serum albumin is a good guide to the severity of chronic liver disease. A healthy liver manufactures plenty of albumin and falling levels of blood albumin show deteriorating liver function.

Globulin protein:

Normal range is 20 - 32g/L or 2 - 3.2g/dL

Blood levels of globulin may be abnormal in chronic liver disease. Elevated levels of globulin proteins in the blood usually mean excessive inflammation in the liver and/or immune system. Very high levels may be seen in some types of cancers.

CHAPTER FIFTEEN

Confessions of a Fat Man
A personal journey from fatty liver disease

An autobiographical essay by Thomas Eanelli MD

Introduction

I have been to hell, and it's not some fiery, scary, raging inferno; rather, it's the feeling of despair and hopelessness you get when you have been devoured and consumed within the belly of an addiction.

- Thomas R. Eanelli MD
www.confessionsofafatman.com

Everyone has a secret. Sure, some people hide their secrets better than others. But make no mistake: we are all flawed in some way or another. I have an eating disorder. Sure, people know I eat too much: it's hard to hide a size 48 waistline and a prodigious appetite.

But that's not my secret.

My secret is that my eating disorder has slowly and insidiously damaged my liver. And even though I walk through life pretending to those around me that all is well, I can assure you: all is not well.

Despite my warm and humorous nature, and despite my reputation as a good physician, patient advocate, father, and friend, I live every day with the knowledge that every time I succumb to my demons and go off my program, I am adding fuel to an already out of control fire.

Sadly, as my story began 40 years ago, many of my health concerns could have been prevented or at least minimized had the traditional medical community been aware of the long-term implications of having a "fatty liver." To make matters worse, I am not alone: far from it.

Due to the global spread of our high fat, highly processed, fast food-based western diet and frenetic, jet-setting lifestyle, fatty liver syndrome has become an epidemic of critical proportions. Indeed, this epidemic is arguably more frightening than the current flu epidemic because it is silent, capricious, and its cure depends on the inner strength and willpower of a historically weak and undisciplined species—one endowed with selective evolutionary predilections toward gluttony. Moreover the until recently near universal misconception that having a fatty liver is a relatively benign condition, incapable of causing terminal damage, still dominates the medical community.

The truth of the matter is that a fatty liver, whether due to too many apple martinis or too much apple pie, can lead to permanent damage known as cirrhosis, which, sadly, can lead to liver failure and death.

Moreover, because a fatty liver has vague or even absent symptomatology up until late stage, and because until recently a large number of doctors habitually dropped the ball and failed to raise an eyebrow at slightly abnormal liver chemistries, many people are still being forced to face a rude awakening. They then will need to make important lifestyle changes, and join me on this difficult and scary journey to reclaim their well being.

Yet there is hope—not just for me, but for all of us who walk the earth hiding this dark and shameful secret.

And that hope is manifested in the work of Dr. Sandra Cabot. Over the course of this story you will get to know a lot about me, probably more than you care to know.

More importantly, however, you will get to know Sandra—

as clinician, self help guru, and health care advocate, but most of all as a person who has dedicated her life to helping people with liver problems.

Sandra is a medical doctor who started her career in the subspecialty of obstetrics and gynecology. She is also, in my mind, the patron saint of fatty liver.

When most people in the medical industry were turning a blind eye to the implications of our sugar-laden, fast-food Western diet, as it relates to the choking and killing of our livers, Sandra was facing the reality of one of the most important, most neglected, and soon to be widespread health problems on this planet.

Sandra saw what few had seen before her: that people can die or become terribly ill simply by neglecting and abusing their livers through their lifestyle choices.

I remember going to my internist after reading Sandra's book and being lectured to and ridiculed on the grounds that her argument lacked a scientific, evidential basis.

As a doctor and a scientist, I am well aware of the need for proper medical studies using randomized trials, i.e. taking matched patient cohorts and studying the effects of different medications or dietary lifestyles in a controlled study, following the subjects over time, and reporting on the different endpoints.

However, in this case the medical community was so oblivious to what was happening in plain sight that it failed to provide prospective data on which to base such studies. So Sandra did what no other doctor had done previously: she risked her medical reputation by venturing into the world of complementary and naturopathic medicine in order to blaze a trail for all of us!

The following testimonial, which I wrote almost ten years ago, recounts how I first came upon Sandra:

A Note of Thanks to Dr. Sandra Cabot
by Thomas R. Eanelli MD

Let me start with a powerful and accurate statement:

Dr. Cabot has literally saved my life!

Words cannot fully express the thanks and gratitude that I feel, not only for her groundbreaking and innovative work on liver cleansing for a healthful life, but, more importantly, for the incredible personal interest, empathy, and involvement that she shows in her patients' progress and happiness.

Please allow me to share something of my incredible story and journey. I am the product of a typically neurotic third-generation Italian American household. We owned a bakery, and both food and love were in abundance. Unfortunately, so were depression and compulsive behavior. As a matter of fact, no member of my family is not obese, alcohol/drug dependent, or a pathological gambler. My father, for example, was an abusive alcoholic who died of cirrhosis at the age of 48, when I was 12. Not coincidentally, I still trace my emotional, nervous binge eating to this horrific period in my life.

After high school my compulsive overeating became uncontrollable, and I passed the 250 pound mark for the first time during my freshman year of college. My weight gain was so logarithmic that I quickly learned the embarrassment and sorrow of stretch marks and the humiliation of patronizing specialty clothing stores. There were brief periods of successful dieting (you name it, I tried it!), but these were always followed by rebound weight gain.

From 1979 until 1985, I weighed between 270 and 350 pounds. My "flaw fatale" was not sweets, but rather salty meats, deep fried foods, pizza, and fast food. My cousin John was my partner in crime, and our "finest moments" make some of the scenes from the movie Fatso eerily realistic. It was not unusual during a binge for us to eat 12 to 14 "equivalents", a term we invented to standardize measurement across different types of food (a hot dog was 1 equivalent, a Big Mac was 1.25 equivalents, etc.). Typically, these sessions would end with us reaching the point of physical illness.

Incredibly, my obesity did not detract from a stellar scholastic career that included a medical degree from a prestigious school, a successful practice, a traditional marriage with three lovely children, strong friendships and a position of honor and respect in my community.

Little did I know, however, that a physiological time bomb in my liver was about to explode!

My medical epiphany took place in 1997, during a business trip to Kansas City. After a 5-hour plane flight, several pieces of pepperoni pizza, ribs, and beer, I went back to my hotel room, undressed, and was horrified to see what stared back at me from the mirror. Instead of a successful 37 year-old man, I saw a 60 year-old, obese, bloated, edematous father of three young children who would be lucky to see their high school graduation, let alone their weddings.

I summoned up the courage to see my internist for the million-dollar work up: blood tests, nuclear scans, stress tests, echocardiogram and cat scans. I'll never forget the conversation we had during our meeting to review the test results: "No problem", he said, "all you have is a fatty liver". At first, I was ecstatic. I was OK, healthy, never mind that I weighed 159 kilograms and my liver enzymes were off the charts. My doctor said I was fine. I could resume my old lifestyle, try to employ moderation, and live to be 100.

But deep in the recesses of my scientifically trained mind something did not sit right. As a matter of fact my abnormal liver function had first been discovered during a routine blood test when I was 20. After the hepatitis screen returned negative, the matter had quickly been dropped.

Why? Suddenly it struck me, harder than a ton of bricks or a Mack truck: I was being railroaded by the mainstream medical community, whose practitioners tell upper middle class suburbanites exactly what they want to hear, and then sign their untimely death certificates with scarcely an afterthought.

It was then that I realized that if I was going to live long enough to see any gray hairs on my head, I would have to take matters into my own hands.

To be fair, I do not wish to be too hard on any one individual. Rather, the blame rests squarely with the medical education system, in which nutritional knowledge is handed out in parsimonious bits and pieces like expensive brandy or caviar at a company Christmas party. However, this reluctance to discuss matters of holistic health or to acknowledge the devastating effects that "bad eating habits" can have on one's physiology was, and remains so pervasive in the mainstream medical community that, much as I needed help, I did not know where to turn.

To my amazement, my exhaustive expedition through the annals of reputable medical literature failed to turn up anything more than a few incidental and vague references to fatty liver (steatosis). Sure, there was a wealth of information about alcoholic cirrhosis, idiopathic biliary—blah, blah, blah, but there was a glaring absence of information regarding the nefarious precursor of a scarred liver that is steatosis. How, I wondered, was the body to know the difference between four Scotch and sodas a night and two greasy, special sauce-laden Big Macs a day, if the end result in either case is fatty accumulation that eventually turns into scar tissue? The answer is that it doesn't, and that realization, too, made me feel as if someone had struck me between the eyes with a 4 x 4.

It turned out that along with all the wonderful gifts that God had given me—brains, Romanesque good looks, charm, charisma—He had likewise given me an Achilles liver.

There are millions of overweight individuals walking this earth with normal hepatic enzymes who are slowly suffocating their livers with fat, but for some reason, I was the one destined to be vulnerable to this poorly defined puzzle of a disease.

In other words, I was in big trouble.

As I had failed outstandingly on every diet known to man, along with hypnosis and acupuncture to boot, it was painfully apparent that a self-directed program would be futile.

My next excursion to good health took me to a fat clinic, where the soup de jour included lackluster liquid, chalky meals, heart damaging amphetamines and a lot of questions about why I hated my mother.

Becoming desperate, I even flew out to San Diego for the annual International Bariatric Surgical meeting to pick up some information about gastric (stomach) bypass and stapling. In doing so I met some wonderful, non-judgmental, sincere, caring people. This is probably because most of the support staff were former patients whose lives had been drastically changed by this operation, and as callous and detached as surgeons are known to be, I found this subset of specialists to be truly concerned and dedicated to using their gifts and skills to try to reconfigure the gastrointestinal tract to mechanically force weight loss to occur.

The downside to such procedures can include not only the inability to consume more than sips and bites of food but also vitamin deficiency issues, malnutrition, dumping syndrome, worsening of fat accumulation in the liver, and operative failure. Nonetheless, I was convinced that this was the way to go, and tentatively booked my case with the world's most experienced key hole (laparoscopic) surgeon, who reportedly could rebuild an engine through a carburetor.

The only caveat I voiced to my surgeon was my refusal

to go on the operating room table weighing 350 pounds. I had seen too many cases of postoperative thrombosis, infection, and pneumonia, and did not want to become another statistic in their morbidity and mortality hospital rounds. I therefore decided to lose a few pounds through diet and exercise to prepare myself for my new life.

Now many people don't believe in karma, kismet, cosmic directives, divine intervention, or even putting pineapple on their pizza, but I do. Thus, it is clear to me that on that fateful day while browsing at the Barnes and Noble superstore in Paramus, New Jersey, God purposely led me to an off-the-beaten-track shelf containing a bright green paperback book entitled **The Liver Cleansing Diet** — written, according to the publisher's blurb, by some Aussie medical doctor named Sandra Cabot.

When I first spotted the title, I literally had to do a double take and force myself out of shock. After all, I had just spent three months in Ivy League medical libraries, logged hundreds of hours on the Internet and joined and contributed to the American Liver Foundation.

I had flown across the country to hear internationally recognized physicians speak about morbid obesity and its inherent health hazards, and all I had discovered about fatty liver disease had been a few abstracts, blank stares, topic changing segues, and off color jokes.

Yet here I was in the sort of chain book store where bibliophiles (book lovers) go to die, lost among racks of the Old New Testament, the New Old Testament, Erma Bombeck meets Tom Clancy, and Kama Sutra for the Double Jointed, and out of left field I had spotted a book that was completely devoted to information about liver health.

My luck was changing.

When I got home, I devoured the book immediately and then re-read it about five times. It was well written, comprehensive, light heartedly illustrated, and easy to follow. It could appeal just as easily to a cosmetologist as to a hepatologist. And the best thing of all was that, for me at least, it told me what to do!

Forget the heart, the brain, and the reproductive tract. Fix the liver and good health will follow.

The most ingenious and helpful aspect of Sandra's book is that it focuses on the body's largest, most vascular, and most metabolically active organ. Paradoxically it is also the organ that is least understood, most often ignored and most grossly underrated—at least in Western tradition—in terms of its importance for weight control, good health and longevity.

Once I began Sandra's program, the weight literally began to melt off me in an eerie, "Wicked Witch of the West gets caught in a summer rain" sort of way.

The change was so drastic and rapid that people began to worry that I had a serious disease, but their concerns quickly vanished when they were unable to reconcile them with the radiant glow of good health and energy that emanated from my inner self.

I couldn't believe how good I felt!

My liver enzymes and cholesterol dropped to almost unimaginably low levels for me. I also restarted the modest exercise program that I had struggled with my whole adult life:

- 30 minutes on the Stairmaster, level 4, 2 times per week
- Circuit around the Nautilus track
- 3 mile run thrown in for good luck every full moon

After only one month I felt as if I were sleepwalking through the once challenging and difficult routine. Indeed, my previous aerobic and athletic barriers started falling faster than Internet stock.

Easy hiking soon led to full gear weekend backpacking trips, which in turn led to section hiking the Appalachian

Trail. Peakbagging mountain excursions summiting small hills in my native New Jersey grew to encompass the more challenging Catskill and Adirondack Mountains of New York, the Green and White Mountains of Vermont and New Hampshire, and ultimately the dizzying heights of Mt. Hood, Mt. Rainier, and their Cascade sisters.

Similarly, three-mile runs turned into five and ten mile races, which soon led to half and then to full marathons and triathlons. Never mind that I usually came in close to last: I was competing in events that I used to dream about. I was grasping life for all it was worth.

Then, last summer, standing on top of Mt. Rainier, I began to cry. My group thought that I was demoralized, hypoxic, and physically exhausted. On the contrary, I was rejuvenated. Each step I took, each muscular contraction, was a celebration of myself. I might as well have been standing on the moon, that's how far I felt I had come.

I was no longer a spectator but a participant.

This is the gift that Dr Sandra Cabot's book has given to me, a gift as miraculous as the birth of a child, an ocean sunset, a field of wildflowers. She gave me—a compulsive, long-suffering overeater and victim of fatty liver disease—a life program that is a literal and tangible fountain of youth! More importantly, this miraculous transformation not only drastically improved my health, energy, and motivation; it also bolstered my self-confidence and helped me to grow in many other positive directions:

- I became more involved as a father once I could get down on my knees and play with my children at eye level. Weekends are now crammed with long walks, bike trips, runs, swims, hikes, rollerblading and skiing.

- I became a more energetic doctor, starting a local cancer survivor group that has touched thousands of lives and has helped raise tens of thousands of dollars for research and philanthropy (www.crocalumni.org).

- I began taking acting classes and participating in community theater.

- Last but not least, I became inspired to follow a lifelong dream and explore myself through creative writing, a dream that I never had the energy or confidence to pursue.

But my story does not end there. It will never end for any compulsive overeater. Like Charlie in Flowers for Algernon, I wake up every morning in a cold sweat out of fear of losing the control and confidence that I have gained. Food is my kryptonite, my enemy. As I painfully observe others who are able to enjoy good food in moderation, and who can treat meals as enjoyable social events, it takes every ounce of strength for me to show restraint.

I would be lying if I said that since I've been on the program I have been completely faithful. There have been many days when I have strayed, or fallen into a lull of complacency. I would stop weighing myself for fear of recognizing the obvious. My clothes would tighten and that paralyzing fear would return. It is at this point that I relax and try not to get angry with myself. Then, I pick up that weathered, overused, bright green book, start from the beginning, and thank God for that Aussie doctor named Sandra Cabot.

How This Book on Fatty Liver Came to Be

Owing to the astonishing power of the Internet, this small testimonial made me better known as a poster boy for fatty liver than I had ever been for the many acts of medical excellence that I humbly believe I have provided to patients in my primary specialty as an oncologist (cancer treatment specialist). I have received calls from frightened people newly diagnosed with fatty liver from South Africa to San Francisco. I even received a call from my seventh grade teacher, who contacted me after reading my testimonial without at first realizing that I had been her student.

Since that time, almost ten years ago, Sandra has been asking me to collaborate with her on a book about fatty liver. And for at least two years, I told her that the first chapter would be heading her way any time now. Yet I hesitated. Why? For one thing, co-authoring a book with Sandra is an opportunity of a lifetime and one that I was not sure I felt qualified to undertake. After all, despite being a medical doctor, my knowledge of liver physiology and clinical hepatology is about as vast as my knowledge of the mating habits of the North American earthworm. With this in mind, how could I co-author a book with one of the most knowledgeable liver people in the world?

In addition, there was the question of privacy versus public exposure and humiliation. Once this book is published, and these words are read, they will be telling the story of an intimate part of my life about which few people know. I couldn't help but think that if my story gets out into the world, the perception that people have of me will be forever changed. I will no longer be known as Dr. Thomas Richard Eanelli, radiation oncologist, but as that guy with the binge eating disorder and the diseased liver.

Lastly and most importantly, however, is the fact that I have been a terrible role model. With most self-help books, including diet programs, the authors are walking, talking, breathing and shining examples of the principles that they preach. I, however, have sometimes squandered the gift and the opportunity of a new and healthy life by failing to stay consistent with the inspired doctrine that got me off the bench and into the game of life.

How can I, a person who has benefited from Sandra's program but who continues to gain and lose ground against his food addiction, make any sort of valid or genuine appeal to help other victims of fatty liver?

To be fair, for the majority of the last ten years I have followed the liver cleansing lifestyle and continued my extreme sporting activities. Yet in no way do I want to misrepresent myself and thereby soil Sandra's reputation—as if, for those who remember the incident, she were Oprah and I was the deceitful author James Fry.

Above all, I think, it is this fear of inauthenticity and contradiction that has kept me from going public with my story. In the end however, my gratitude toward Sandra and her work, along with my desire to feel well and also to help other people in the same boat, won out and motivated me to write these words.

You see, I have felt the sting of fear and despair when I was told about my liver problem by an ambivalent and uninformed medical system, and I have felt the thrill and relief of being able to reverse my fortune. I have been up the mountain and down the mountain, both literally and figuratively. Yet I truly believe that the only reason I am here today is because of Sandra's book and because I have never completely drifted from the core elements of her healthy liver program.

In addition, I know that there are people like me out there who are suffering from an addiction that is causing their livers to die. And even though I'm not perfect and I lead a sloppy and altogether human life, I think that my story has potential benefits for those people who are finding out that their livers are choking with fat - and who want to know what they can do about it.

CHAPTER ONE
The Sins of Our Fathers

My liver story dates back to 1956, four years before I was born, and involves a man whom I never met. It is an ugly story that I'm sure will be as hard to read as it was to write.

But it is an important story that has the potential—if fully and honestly told—to positively impact others' lives.

First, I as the author need to establish a covenant with you, the reader. Only by sharing my inner demons and embarrassing secrets can I gain the trust that I need from you to look within your own life to come to grips with your own personal liver story, whether that story involves hepatitis or excessive drinking, drug or eating habits. Besides, I know from experience how skeptical you may have become: I have read many self-help books written by people with Ivy League degrees in hepatology or with "expertise" in eating disorders or addiction, but who lack the personal experience to make their work relevant or really connected to the lives of others. That's not to say that a writer or clinician has to have the problem in order to help cure the problem, but in buying a book and devoting time to reading it, you want to feel confident that it actually pertains to your situation.

For example, as a food addict, I once read a book by a woman with a Ph.D. in eating disorders who attempted to relate to me on the basis that once upon a time she had been around eight pounds overweight (there was no mention of a fatty liver), and she had the dickens of a time trying to get back to "normal." Not to belittle that author's problems, but I can and sometimes do gain around eight pounds on a weekend bender! Thus, from my point of view, this well-educated and probably well-intentioned author spent 300 pages trying to help me develop strategies for a condition that she did not truly understand. More fool me, of course, that I bought her book...

It is therefore crucial that, for the purposes of our journey through this book, we expand our frame of reference when it comes to how we think about fatty liver. We must be keenly aware that there are many roads to this disease, and that each person's story is unique. In fact, we should also be aware that the majority of the so-called experts may have grossly underestimated the true impact of this epidemic. Of course, I hope and pray that the problem is less severe than I portray it to be, and I would gladly be proved wrong and be chased around the countryside by liver experts and health academics carrying pitchforks, calling me a heretic and scare-monger.

Unfortunately, however, it is more likely that we stand at the epicenter of a tsunami of food-related steatosis (the technical term for fatty liver disease or FLD), which I believe is becoming so prolific that it deserves its own moniker: non-alcoholic steatohepatitis, or NASH to its victims like you and me. And if you think our livers care whether the fat came from alcohol, food, drugs or hepatitis C, or that the type of cirrhosis we become vulnerable to is any less deadly, you are gravely mistaken.

Please be aware, too, that death by cirrhosis is not a pretty sight. If you don't die bedridden and yellow, with a swollen belly encased in tortuous enlarged veins, with your hands flapping and your mind confused in an ammonium-induced brain inflammation, then you die from the proverbial GI bleed, which took the lives of both my father and grandfather. And, as hard as it will be to hear, it is crucial for you to know their stories, as well as my story, in order to be aware of the true potential destruction a liver disorder can impart on its unsuspecting host.

My liver story, then, began with my grandfather's death four years before I was born. To this day, I wonder what my grandfather was thinking as he gasped his last breath while anxious junior doctors scurried about trying unsuccessfully to pump pints of fresh packed red blood cells into his circulatory system faster than he was losing his own blood from a "bleeding ulcer."

The term "bleeding ulcer" or gastrointestinal (GI) bleed is used as a catch-all label behind which sleep-deprived hospital staff hide, as they tried to assuage the grief of family members whom they deem too fragile to hear the truth about hemorrhaging esophageal veins, a result of end-stage cirrhosis. The thought that their loved ones died from a bowery bum disease would certainly be a hard pill to swallow, one that would require a lengthy and empathetic explanation for it to be palatable. Sadly, time and empathy are both commodities of which medical staff rarely has much to spare.

So, instead we settled on this mutually agreeable and comfortable diagnosis, a détente of sorts, such that grieving families would not have to be hit over the head with the socially awkward truth that Daddy or Uncle Bill were indeed raging drunks, and we, on the staff side, could sign off on the death certificate and maybe get some sleep...

I wonder if my father was there when his father died. More importantly, I wonder if he knew the implications of his father's death, as I now understand those of my father's death.

At the age of 31, my father was already a full-blown alcoholic whose liver was beginning to accumulate the fat that would later lead to the full blown scarring known as cirrhosis. Eventually, the liver becomes scarred beyond recognition and is unable to support the gallons of venous blood flowing through it returning back to the right side of the heart. This, in turn, causes a gradual increase in venous pressure, forcing new tributaries and routes through veins such as the hemorrhoidal, umbilical, and—you guessed it—esophageal systems, which were never designed to handle that much strain.

Sadly, the physiological effects of his alcoholism were not my father's only problem and over-indulgence was not his only fault. By the time I was seven, my mother and I had already had to escape his drunken tirades by retreating to a small one bedroom apartment in a low-income block in Paterson New Jersey. My father, for his part, was subsequently exiled to a sad and lonely room in the downtown Alexander Hamilton Hotel.

By the time I was eight, he had become a mere shell of a man, and any time that I did spend with him he spent sitting on a barstool. Mind you, the bar scene in the 1960s was nothing like it is today. There was nothing glamorous or exotic about Sandy's Bar, or about any other Paterson gin mill. They were dirty, dark, dank places filled with pathetic and addicted drunks who, like my father, had for the most part gotten themselves thrown out of their homes and, effectively, out of their own lives.

Although my father was no better a man than any other alcoholic sitting on those stools, the level of talent and potential that were frittered away as a result of his destructive addiction truly set him apart. No one who knew him and spoke to me of him, either when he was alive or since, has failed to mention to me what a great shame and waste this was. A gifted pianist, his talent was nurtured in classical style by his aunt, but took shape in the pre-war jazz clubs of the neighborhood. He was so good, in fact, that he was recruited out of high school by big band legend Gene Krupa, and was soon accompanying and arranging for Mel Torme and Peggy Lee. He was at the top of his profession, traveling the world and rubbing shoulders with the rich and famous entertainers of the time.

Unfortunately, one of the occupational hazards of the entertainment industry is substance abuse, and I am given to understand that my father's habit was legendary, even by Hollywood standards. Yet I never really knew when his fall came about or why. Some people tell me that being drafted into the war robbed his career of its momentum. Others blame his decision to go to college after the war. Personally, I rather suspect that the problem was not any specific trigger but the cumulative effect of his lifestyle: as time went on and his liver became sicker and sicker, his desire to produce and succeed became less important to him than feeding the beast.

The saddest thing for me is that I only heard stories of his glory days. I never knew the funny and gregarious man who was always described as the life of the party. And I only got to hear him play the piano a handful of times.

The man I knew as my father was the one whose liver and inner light were both already dead. I don't remember him playing Vegas, or doing sessions with Nat King Cole. I only remember him begging for gigs in run-down, second-class joints that did not deserve his skills or talent.

By the time I was nine, my dad was bringing alcohol into the schools where he taught. He kept his small stash discreetly hidden and concealed its traces expertly with breath freshener aerosols. But there was always the mother load carefully hidden under the front seat of his third-hand Oldsmobile, to which he resorted for hourly refills.

By the time I turned ten, his urine had turned brown and I knew that he was sick.

By the time I turned eleven, his urine had turned black and I knew that he was gone. It was only a matter of time.

I was only a kid, and I should not have been privy to the color of an old man's bodily waste. But by then my father had lost all semblance of personal pride. He had also lost the physical ability to snap himself out of the night's drunken stupor, even if it was only to relieve himself in the proper place. So, instead, he lined the window ledge above the worn, stained patent leather couch with preserve jars — not cheap, screw top jars but the old-fashioned type, with thick, etched glass depicting happy winter scenes complete with horse drawn carriages and plump cheeked, laughing children. They sealed hermetically with built-in lids and matching rubber O-rings. They could keep things fresh for hundreds of years if necessary, and I found it unbearably sad that these hand-blown works of craftsmanship, once dignified to contain freshly picked, plump red tomatoes or sugary sweet apricots, should now find themselves defiled with diseased urine.

At dusk the jars sat empty, lined up like prison guards keeping sentry over the bugs that foraged for crumbs in the dark. By dawn, however, the jars would be filled to the brim with foamy amber poison. If I got up at just the right time, when the sun had risen to just the right spot, beams of light would reflect off the cheap, dirty vinyl blinds in such a way that the glass would glow with a brilliant supernatural phosphorescence and animate strange, otherworldly clumps of matter. These particles would flow chaotically through the liquid, as if performing a dance of joy at being freed from their corporeal imprisonment.

At first, the jars intrigued me. Did this really come out of my father's body? Why was the color of the pee the same color as his whiskey? Did the booze make his kidneys too drunk and lazy to turn it yellow? Silly thoughts, I know. But my powers of reasoning were still in development.

By the time I was twelve, the superintendent had found his naked body coiled in a heap in the bathroom, drowned in the blood of his own GI bleed. We buried him on a cold wet day in November 1972. My entire grade school class walked in the rain, all the way from St. Gerard's School on West Broadway to St. Michael's Church, which was in the Little Italy section of downtown. I will never forget the stares of pity that I received as they passed me, sitting in the black funeral home sedan—made all the worse because it reflected back at me the gnawing sense of self-pity that I had secretly harbored for as long as I could remember.

Growing up with a serious alcoholic in the immediate family is like living on death row. One goes through the motions of daily life and tries to keep up a pretense of hope, but all the time one is almost eager for the final day to come. While most of my friends and cousins looked forward to things like Christmas and vacations, he and I just were. We had an unspoken understanding. He would go to work and I would go to school. He would pick me up on Mondays and Wednesdays after school and we would hang out either at a bar or at a place that had a bar, such as the bowling alley. Some Fridays I would sleep over, but he would pass out before dark, leaving me alone with my brewing anxiety.

It is to those moments in my father's tiny room that I trace the beginnings of my eating disorder and the foundation of my destiny as a third generation prince of liver disease. But instead of booze, I found food.

For me, using food instead of drugs or liquor to calm my fears and insecurities was a no brainer. After all, I did grow up in an Italian immigrant family in which the supreme emphasis was on food. And when I say food, I mean the most awesome and delicious peasant ambrosia ever to come out of a mortal's kitchen.

My grandfather, a former bakery apprentice from Naples, ran a pastry shop on Market Street in Paterson. This establishment not only provided him and much of the family with its livelihood, it gave me virtually unlimited access to the world's greatest cannolis, spumoni, homemade gelato, cookies and rum cake—the latter accounting for the only alcohol that I have ever knowingly consumed.

All our meals were excessive, but Sundays and holidays were particularly gluttonous. My grandmother's Sunday sauce was so good that it became known as "red gold," and its secret recipe was her culinary pride and her family's indulgent joy. The meatballs would start sizzling in the frying pan before breakfast, which would include the few "naked" (sauceless) ones that we could steal without being hit with grandmother's wooden spoon or cursed in her Neopolitan dialect. The rest of the kindred meats, like the sausages and brazole, would all converge and cavort together like buoys bobbing in a sea of maroon in an industrial size European iron cauldron that could only be lifted by my muscle bound uncles—or by my grandmother herself, who was every bit as strong and hairy.

Holiday meals were outstandingly gluttonous, beginning with mountains of antipasto overflowing with olives, artichokes, roasted peppers, salted meats and sharp cheeses. Then came the pasta and meat sauce—and, as if that weren't enough, there were usually two or three American style roasts, like beef, turkey, veal or lamb, all accompanied with their respective side dishes. Dessert followed, with representations from all categories of bakery fare, and the food fest would continue through late-night snacks of sandwiches made from the leftovers of the feast.

Basically, I was living on a non-stop, landlocked buffet style cruise ship!

I could go on and on about all the great food I've consumed, but I'm sure by now you get the idea—besides, I'm getting hungry just thinking about it, which is a bad thing (we'll return later to the issue of food fantasies).

More important than what I was eating—or even how much—was what the food experience brought to me: a brief feeling of release and comfort in a world devoid of parental love and protection. It was a way of saying "stuff you" to my father and his drinking. It was a way of me saying "stuff you" to a lost childhood. It was a way of saying "stuff you" to any normal development of self-love that would have been the proper avenue of functional growth for a ten year old kid. Basically food became my savior and my assassin, my identity and my estrangement, my companion and my nemesis.

I used to visit my father's grave often, riding my bike the two miles from the tenement to the cemetery. His headstone is five rows down, one stone in. Five and one. I needed those numbers to remind me of where he was buried. I know it sounds crazy now. After all, how hard could it be to find your own father's grave? Shouldn't there be some sort of familial sonar that would work even if the paternal beacon were buried six feet underground? But I kept getting lost among the gravestones, and I desperately needed to come up with a system to orient myself within this field of granite shrines. Rows of headstones lined up like West Point cadets, dull gray yet stoic, eerily silent yet curiously animated. Most had etchings of angels or crosses, immaculate Mary's, and innocent Saints, hands together in prayer, with beatific arcs around their heads, praying for all the dead sinners.

I used to make up stories about these dead people. The stories would be mainly imagined from the ethnicities of the names of the deceased, as well as on the number of years that he or she had spent on earth (a pretty easy calculation based on subtracting the year of death from the year of birth, but good mathematical practice for a young lad), and on the year of death (which, in turn, was good history practice, since in my imagination I would relate the dates to banner plague years like 1918, and to notable periods of warfare like 1941 to 1945, 1955 to 1958, and 1965 to 1971...). Perhaps, for example, Joseph Catchatori, age 82, had died face down in his bowl of Sunday rigatoni from a massive heart attack. Or maybe Emma Webster, age 66, had been mangled by a drunk 16-year-old hit-and-run driver while taking a lonely summer stroll down some secluded rural road. And, most certainly, Pfc. Douglas Baldini had died with merciful speed after the bayonet of the camouflaged 12-year-old Viet Kong guerrilla soldier plunged deeply into his left ventricle.

Deep inside I knew that my daydreaming was just a way to catapult my otherwise overwhelmed and numb mind as far away as possible from my gnawing grief. (To make matters worse, my father and I shared the same name, which made it a creepy affair for a 12-year-old boy to see his own name on a stone slab proclaiming death.) I also knew that there was no pretense of heroic or romantic sacrifice that could be associated with my father's death: no courageous assaults on an enemy pillbox while 50 caliber bullets made Swiss cheese out of his guts and no blood dripping from slashed wrists for lost love. But lack of sacrifice does not exclude the potential of redemption, his or mine. One just has to know where to find it. And for us, the seed of redemption comes hidden within the tragedy of my father's death and the irony of my own life.

Still, I trace the roots of my food addiction directly to the trauma of my childhood, and this awareness is not new for me. So it was that I spent many angry years harboring submerged hatred and anger over my father's frailties and imperfections. How could he let himself be controlled by this addiction? How could he subject me to such danger? If he really loved me, could he not have easily stopped drinking? As time passed, my questions sharpened rather than dulled, my inability to forgive created a huge chip on my shoulder, and my attitude of entitlement tarnished all of my relationships. The older I got, the more childishly I behaved because I was consumed with jealousy and unhappiness. It didn't matter that my father had been dead three times longer than the number of years we had shared together, I remained an incomplete, self-hating and electively disenfranchised person—that is, until I finally began to be aware of my own liver issues, which were, as the rhyme goes, "self inflicted because [I was] addicted".

To this day, I remain in shock that it took so long for me to put the pieces together. Yes, it is true that before I encountered Dr Sandra Cabot, I did not receive what I believe to be adequate medical guidance. And yes, it is true that the damage done to my psyche was so deep that it took decades of self help, introspection and painful professional counseling for me to reach the point where I cannot only forgive my father, but can actually empathize with and relate to him, as well as to any other addicted individual, regardless of their choice of poison. But I should have known better, not because I had a medical degree (as it turned out, my trust in Western medicine was a liability in this case), rather, I should have realized that I had been so busy blaming everyone else for my problems that I lacked the necessary ability to take responsibility for my own actions. It wasn't until I read Sandra's book that I was able to see the big picture.

In essence, the information that Sandra has been shouting for years to get into the public's hands has both humbled and liberated me from the shackles of self-righteousness. I now recognize that, like someone stuck in quicksand, flailing in self-pity only pulls you further down a deep hole. Let's face it: everyone has a story, equally, if not more, compelling than mine. But we have to get over it, whatever it is, before we can move forward and achieve inner peace—and provided it's not too late, good liver health and longevity!

Maybe then, my father's life can be significant after all. For it is precisely the damage that his addiction did to his body, to his talent and to his mind, as well as the profound impact it had on those around him, that can serve as a great motivator to bring attention to and help us control our bad habits, addictions and resultant liver disease. That, at any rate, is the theme of this book, and that, as I see it, is my father's redemption.

To tell you the truth, not a week goes by that I don't wake up in a cold sweat because of a recurring dream about my own GI bleed, collapsed in a cheaply tiled bathroom, suffocating in my own blood. Yet since I met Sandra and came to terms with my father's life and death, the dreams are becoming less frightening and less paralyzing. Now, they serve more to motivate and inspire me to remain constantly vigilant in my personal journey and in my battle with food—and, more importantly, to make me more forgiving of my own human weaknesses and imperfections, and a more loving and accepting human being.

How I know this to be true is simple. My father's gravestone states that he lived for 48 years. I am 49 years old as I write this. Because of Sandra, I am in unchartered waters. Despite all the damage I have done to myself, I am still here—maybe not thin as a beanpole, maybe still succumbing to a binge here and there, but still in the game, raising my three children in person and writing my story to help others sort through their own liver traumas. That is my redemption.

CHAPTER TWO

The Liver Is My Life

Two pixies delivered dinner to my room last night. It didn't matter that the girls were sweet, cute and petite—they could just as well have been Belarusian heavyweight wrestlers. The point is that it took two human beings to carry my dinner: two grilled cheese sandwiches with French fried potatoes, two half pound bacon cheeseburgers with more French fried potatoes, dill pickles, onions, lettuce and tomatoes, bread pudding with ice cream and chocolate cake. All of these items were imprisoned in individual domed serving trays to keep in the heat or cold, depending on the course. I also ordered four beverages to give the impression that the mountain of food was going to be divvied up between four normal adults instead of consumed by one individual with a binge eating disorder.

Sometimes I go through a whole series of dramatic overtures to lessen the indignity and embarrassment brought on by the incredulous or critical stares of clerks, room service personnel, fast food grill masters and doughnut makers, not to mention their wise cracks. Often, I turn on the shower and leave the bathroom door open just enough to give the impression that there's another person in the room. As a responsible ecologically minded individual, however, I usually conserve water and instead make up an elaborate story such as, "I'm expecting colleagues for dinner", or "I will shortly be hosting a small reunion of the 33rd Cavalry Regiment". Usually, though, these ruses fail, and I can see (or imagine) that the person can't wait to leave the room so they can tell the rest of Seattle or Denver what a great bleeping pig he or she just met in the hotel room. All I can do is tip over-generously in a futile attempt to buy the person's silence and bid farewell knowing (or imagining) that I have once again achieved infamy in some food service worker's circle of friends.

Luckily because of Sandra and her program, these binges no longer occur with the frequency that they once did. In fact, if they did, I would not be here to write this book.

Sometimes I know what sets off the binges, like when I find myself outside my home environment, alone in an unfamiliar city, stressed and tired from ten hours or so of professional conference sessions. Other times I don't even understand it myself. Nevertheless, I am keenly aware that whatever fat has been laid down in my liver is the just desserts of my own overindulgence.

Personal accountability is the cornerstone of maturity. Thus, harsh as is my criticism of the denial and lack of interest that have surrounded the phenomenon of fatty liver, I cannot and do not blame my doctors for my own particular problem. What's more, I see my condition as not simply a life-threatening personal problem but also an opportunity to help others. As I mentioned in my testimonial in this book's introduction, the first inkling that I had, that anything was wrong with my liver, came in the summer of 1982, after I graduated from college and before I entered medical school. At that time, routine blood screening revealed elevated liver enzymes, but a negative hepatitis test sadly put an end to further explanation. A few years later, another abnormality, the presence of urobilirubin (bile) was detected in my urine, but again ignored. Finally, in the late 1990s, my liver malfunction indicators went through the roof, and despite my internist's lack of concern, my radar antennae was up for good.

Of all people, it was a pathologist—that is, a physician who studies disease and determines cause of death—who tore back the curtain and made me see the writing on the wall. Schuyler Newman is an intelligent and compassionate physician whom I am proud to call my friend. He is a throwback in the sense that he remains collegial and dignified despite the dog-eat-dog environment surrounding the life of today's physician. He is happy in what he does and good at it, does not slander other doctors, does not advertise his skills, and is always happy to answer a question and go the extra mile to help a patient or colleague. It Is because of Schuyler and his willingness to walk me through the pathological basis of the war going on within my body's largest internal organ that I began my journey of inquiry. However, I had first to absorb the new information, and this took some time. After all, what Schuyler told me amounted to the instant ownership of a disease that I did not know existed as such, let alone know that I had it, and although few doctors had any expertise in this disease, it possessed the potential to kill.

It is fair to say that I have no recollection of leaving Schuyler's office. As a matter of fact, I have very little recollection of the next ten days because I experienced the shock and mortification that one feels when one is told for the first time that one is not as healthy as one thinks—not even close. Along with this, naturally, came the overwhelming fear of dying and leaving my young children without a father.

It's funny how the mind turns inward when we experience shocking events. I have been told that flashbacks are common, and mine took me back to first-year anatomy classes in medical school. Our class had developed a method in which students would take turns recording and transcribing the lectures and distributing them to the rest of the class. This way each student only had to take copious notes a few times each semester, and at all other times we could expect to receive clear, typewritten summaries in our mailboxes within 48 hours of the professor's talk. Often, in our transcriptions, we would try to outdo each other with wit and humor as a way of lessening the pressure of having to process an inconceivable amount of hard-core scientific information. So wouldn't you know that when my turn came, the lecture was about, what else: the liver! I signed the transcription as follows: "Respectfully submitted by Thomas 'the liver is my life' Eanelli". For some reason, this method of signing one's name to a transcription caught on, and soon many of my classmates were playing off my template; naturally my favorite being, Al "Tom Eanelli is my life" Zacharia.

These words of student wit are amusing to recall, but in my post-diagnosis haze I remained transfixed, stuck like a bug in amber in a moment from long ago, frozen in time in a cavernous lecture hall in Piscataway, New Jersey, while memories of classmates and teachers, buildings and labs, white coats and formaldehyde, washed over me. I thought how utterly absurd and surreal it was that the liver had indeed become my life, that on the brink of my fourth decade of life it was now unlikely to be a car, a bolt of lightning, cancer, heart disease, a stroke, or even a jealous husband that would be the death of me, it would be my flipping liver! And to make matters worse, just about everything I knew about the liver I had learned while transcribing that anatomy lecture twenty years earlier. In other words, I was between the proverbial rock and hard place, up the creek without a paddle, or shit out of luck—pick your favorite cliché...

One of the funny things about being a doctor is that it's sort of like skipping to the last page of a mystery novel and knowing the ending before anyone else. And although I have always been curious about certain other careers—such as a race car driver, astronaut, or actor—I have always retained the notion that being a doctor gives a person a unique power: not so much a power over life or death (though one can't say that to a trauma surgeon at a cocktail party!), but rather a power akin to that of fictional detective heroes like Sherlock Holmes. For example, I might find myself on the subway, in a mall, or at my kids' soccer game, and I'll be able to pick out the people with Graves' disease, emphysema, or alcoholism. If someone has had a stroke, I can easily tell you what part of his or her brain has been affected and how badly. Moreover, as an oncologist, I know at a glance what type of chemotherapy the young hairless woman hiding behind the turban has been receiving, I can tell who has been treated with acute head and neck radiation by the residual markings or skin reactions, and I can recognize those who have graduated from the program with the gift of "cottonmouth", by the tell-tale water bottle accessory.

Even more damning is the knowledge of how long a person has to live, just from hearing a few sentences of his or her history or reading a few lines of a pathology report. But what happens when the doctor becomes the patient—when the bell tolls for thee? That was the scary, uncharted sea into which I had sailed. I was making the transition from doctor to patient, from sage to simpleton, from god to mortal. And let me tell you, it was not fun, especially since I was joining a cohort of patients who lacked support groups or even a recognized subspecialty to give them insight, hope, or courage.

Despite my new role and resultant despair, I found a measure of virtue in conceding my mortality. With the vantage point from the other side of the exam table came a sort of nobility born of humility. I was now a patient, not the doctor. Now it was I asking the questions instead of answering them. And it was I who had a vested interest in my fat-laden liver. Thrown into the lions' den, I had become an active participant and a personal advocate, which was quite different from my usual role of all-knowing health care provider seated comfortably in the cozy chair of detachment.

In the 1991 Touchstone Pictures film, The Doctor, directed by Randa Haines, William Hurt plays an arrogant surgeon who is brimming with talent, knowledge and experience but extremely short on empathy. When his throat becomes cancerous the tables are turned and Hurt's character experiences the fear and humility inflicted by doctors like himself. Although I am no huge fan of the movie, I believe that the premise carries an important message for doctors about walking a mile or two in their patients' shoes. This theme is brought home when the title character has his clinical students switch roles with their patients in order to achieve a true understanding of and connection to what it feels like to be sick, hurt and scared.

In the movie the students were lucky to have the importance of such an experience brought home to them early in their careers. But the truth is we all get a turn on the other side of the table sooner or later. The only question is how will we handle it? Being a good patient and handling one's illness intelligently and with dignity requires more than just learning how to be empathetic and humble, or how to feel comfortable sitting on an examination table. It also requires a mindset that allows one to look at one's life and habits in a realistic and truthful way. As doctors, however, we are usually so busy looking at minutiae—and so devoid of introspection—that our thought process, as it relates to our own conduct is comically inaccurate.

For many of us who overeat, there is a tremendous disconnect between the number of calories that we think we are consuming and the number of calories that we actually consume. This discrepancy is not unlike the chasm of covert sneakiness—often as wide as the Grand Canyon—that yawns between imagination and reality for the alcoholic and the drug addict. In all cases, the unifying factor for addictive, self-destructive personality types is the spectre of denial that masks the severity of harm that will surely come our way if we do not stop feeding the beast.

Luckily, if one finally is shocked back to normality, there is the grand realization that one doesn't need a medical degree to evaluate one's own life rationally—much the same way an actuary evaluates probable longevities for insurance companies, based on known facts. Take for instance a vegetarian who keeps his or her weight under control, has no unhealthy addictions, and follows a cardio-aerobically healthy lifestyle. One need not be a doctor or an actuary to reason that, absent any heinous genetic malformation or major traumatic incident, such a person is likely to live well into his or her 80s or beyond, whereas the unfortunate majority, myself included, are more or less self-destructive, in some cases even needing a sledgehammer blow, to wake us up to the years or even decades that we are taking off our potential lifespan.

Take the diabetic whose blood sugars remain out of control for decades; this causes his or her small blood vessels to basically close up, resulting in blindness, neuropathy and multi-organ failure and limb amputations. Take the post-stroke hypertensive no longer able to walk or talk; such a person may often be seen lying shrivelled and contracted in a nursing home bed because he or she refused to take the prescribed medication and stop smoking. Take the person with high cholesterol and triglycerides whose daily diet includes a breakfast of pop tarts, a lunch of cheese burgers, Snickers bars and sweet soda, and a dinner of fettuccini alfredo or some equally high carbohydrate concoction. Such a person's blood is as thick as molasses, and his or her coronary arteries are as clogged as an old rusty drain. Take me, the binge eater and food addict, who has spent an entire lifetime feeding his insecurities and neuroses with Big Macs and Wendy's Triples. We are the people you read about who die suddenly in midlife - we are there one day and gone the next! And everyone asks, "But why?" We are the people who leave our children parentless, and everyone says, "What a sin." We are the people who squander our talents and God-given gifts, and everyone says "What a pity!"

I believe, however, that there is an alternative to dying young. If I did not, I would be traveling the country on a "diners, drive-ins, and dives farewell jag" rather than writing this book. The hope that I have learned to feel, rests on a great many pairs of shoulders, and all should be acknowledged here: Dr Sandra Cabot, who has shouted from the mountaintop the true danger of fatty liver in order to help others make the vital changes that are necessary for us to live long and healthy lives; the many other researchers who have dedicated their lives to eradicating fatty liver; and the many patient, empathetic professionals who are trained and skilled in treating addictions. In addition, my hope rests on the metaphorical shoulders of the considerable restorative powers of the liver itself, as well as on those of the ability that we all have deep down inside to conquer our own fears and to curb our self-destructive behaviors.

Now, when it comes to conquering fears, I'll readily admit that if I were a character from the Wizard of Oz, I would be the Cowardly Lion. But remember: even the Cowardly Lion found his courage in the end. And if I—true namesake of the archetypal skeptic, Doubting Thomas—can find hope and courage and can learn to believe in myself again, then I believe that there is hope for all of us.

True to my nature and my name, however, my initial reaction to my diagnosis was to follow the way of the ostrich: I stuck my head in the sand and continued to binge. I was caught up and sucked into a self-perpetuating vortex that was powered by an irrational notion that I was destined to follow the fate of my grandfather and my father and to suffer an untimely death from ruptured enlarged esophageal veins—a fate that would end with me lying in a bloody, bloated heap on some cheaply tiled, garden apartment bathroom floor.

To my credit, food addictions are not the easiest of monkeys to pry from your back. Food as a general means of providing fuel and nutrition is a good thing. As a matter of fact, great food prepared lovingly can serve as the center point of family and social life. Indeed, some anthropologists believe that the hunt, the kill, and the preparation of game, cemented primitive clans together and spearheaded human socialization and the development of human intelligence. At the same time however, as much as we think that we can distance ourselves from our barbaric forebears, there remains an evolutionary echo, deep within the recesses of our DNA, that tells us that gluttony is good—that we had better eat up while food is abundant and competition low, lest one day we must face a famine unprepared.

Even in our presumably enlightened—or at least educated—post-modern Western world, quantity sells better than quality. The endless "all you can eat" buffets are no longer confined to cruise ships and casinos. In addition, the lines are typically longest at the restaurants that are known for providing huge portions at reasonable prices. And the differential is not always along the lines of wealth versus poverty. After all, what could remind one more of Neanderthal campfires roasting wooly mammoth steaks than the up-market ethnic steakhouse where servers in colorful livery saunter through the aisles carrying skewered slabs of meat ready to be carved at tableside?

Indeed, accessibility is an issue, but its effect is probably the reverse of what one might intuit or find to have been the case a few decades ago. After all, most reasonably populous areas today boast plentiful 24/7 super-duper markets, diners and restaurants representing almost every ethnic cuisine. Forty years ago a block was thought chic if it had a pizzeria and a Chinese kitchen. Today, Chinese food has regionalized, Japanese food is ubiquitous, and there is wide penetration of Thai, Indian, Mediterranean, Mexican, gourmet Italian, peasant Italian, French, Malaysian, Afghani, Ethiopian and

Peruvian bistros, not to mention the gazillions of donut/ ice cream, one-stop, fatten-up stations and caramel latte, yuppie, wannabee Starbuckoriums. Sure, some of the latter are priced to exclude more than a few ordinary Joes, but overall the result is that even the poor and working classes today have vast and dangerous access to food that is often gluttonous by its very nature (I mean the high fat, high-carbohydrate and fatty liver-inducing varieties), and in any case decadent in the excessive amounts that can be easily, quickly and inexpensively consumed.

To make matters worse, the postmodern world is tremendously complex and difficult to maneuver, and it is little wonder that neuroses and personality disorders continue to multiply. Indeed, my childhood story of abuse and alcoholism is a fairy tale compared to the nightmares that some of my addicted friends have survived. But no matter what number the story rates on the horror show Richter scale, the bottom line is that our fractured psyches will fuel the fires of our addictions, and in the case of food, it is available, accessible, and, in fact, unavoidable.

Unavoidable! Let us dissect and tease apart this concept. Now, before I start, I want to state categorically that I make no pretense of acting as judge and jury when it comes to dictating a top ten list of the most heinous things to be addicted to. Who am I to say that being addicted to food is worse than being addicted to drugs or booze or crack or sex or gambling? I am addicted to food and I suffer a pain from this addiction that defies mere words, yet I have no desire to drink anything stronger than Spanish coffee or to put any of my hard-earned money on the nose of a slow horse. Nevertheless, I am extremely empathetic and appreciative of the plight of such addicts, and I share their pain. Therefore, it would be extraordinarily pedantic and cavalier to say that the food path is the most circuitous path. But I will say this: there is no way to avoid food. It is truly unavoidable. As much of a struggle as it is for an alcoholic to walk past a bar, and as much restraint as it must take for a drug addict to decline a fix, they do not have to dip into the kettle of their kryptonite. Conversely, that is exactly what a food addict has to do on a daily basis. Thus, however else one might compare the pain and exigencies of various addictions, it is a fact that we food addicts must dip into the fateful well—one that society and "progress" have turned into a veritable cornucopia—multiple times a day and draw our hands out again by our own power of will, trying to keep within reasonable parameters of quantity. That's like telling a raging alcoholic that in order to live, he or she must drink, one or two ounces of spirits three times each day, yet never shall he or she partake of that third ounce at any one sitting, or pass the six-ounce per day aggregate limit, lest they die. Extend the analogy to cover other addictive substances and I think you'll agree that, were this the case, a heck of a lot of "recovered" or "recovering" addicts would be seen stumbling into their 12 step meetings drunk, stoned and wondering what went wrong!

So it was no wonder that my shift from doctor to patient put me in a tizzy. Not only did it come out of nowhere, not only did no one at the time know much about fatty liver, but now I had to face my food addiction head on or face mortal damage to my liver. Every day I was expected to micromanage every little thing that I put into my mouth. Every single day I was expected to say "No" to foods that had been my staples for 40 years. Every single day I had to face the ghosts of my heritage. Not surprisingly, I went deep into the throws of a full-blown depressive episode.

For months I went through the motions of life. I went to work, I played with the kids and I did the holiday circuit. Throughout this time, I ate everything in my path—no fast food joint stood a chance of avoiding my patronage: McDonald's, Burger King, Wendy's, Taco Bell, Pizza Hut, Arby's—and, of course, the man I trusted most: Colonel Sanders of Kentucky Fried Chicken fame! Yet the ability to derive any enjoyment or satisfaction from even the grandest events of life evaded me. I was among the walking dead—too afraid to die, too afraid to live.

The phenomenon of survival has been written about extensively—specifically, the question of what type of person, when exposed to a horrendous ordeal such as a plane crash, shipwreck or other epic misadventure, is most likely to survive, and which type of person is most likely to die. Basically, the survivors are the ones who keep their cool, stay calm and attentive, continue to problem solve, remain confident, and, above all else, can even retain a sense of humor. Non-survivors, however, lose their equanimity, panic, become confused, unable to think straight and resign themselves to their own death. In other words, if my arm got stuck between two boulders in a remote wilderness and I were alone, I would not be the one who self-amputates using his Swiss army knife and walks out alive; rather, I would be the one found with what's left of me dangling from the crevice.

The secret, I believe, is to know who one is, be okay with that, and develop ways to navigate around the holes in one's character and find its capabilities. Take, for instance, the near tragedy of NASA's failed Apollo 13 mission to land on the moon in 1970. When things went bad and the CO_2 levels began to rise, NASA engineers did not have the luxury of reinventing the equipment that was available to the astronauts. Instead, they had to work with what was already on board, retrofitting odds and ends to create new, usable filters and other devices so that the mission could limp home safely. Fortunately, the astronauts were highly trained and probably natural survivors as well; but most of us are not, and we have to emulate the engineers on the ground: use the bits and pieces of God-given talent and hard-won experience that we have, and fit those pieces together well enough to get past our deficiencies and to overcome the pitfalls that life throws in our path.

With this in mind, it is helpful to consciously maintain a cache of resources to be cobbled together into a life raft or safety net in times of need—which can be every day as well as in moments of special crisis. I have already told you how important Sandra's work has been for me, and I try at least once a week to skim my oft-highlighted copies of her liver books to keep me inspired and focused on the do's and the don'ts of good liver health.

I also have the particular honor of working with cancer patients every day. Let me tell you something: if you ever find yourself in the clutches of self-pity and despair, I urge you to speak to a cancer survivor.

There is a power and peacefulness in knowing that life does not grant one any guarantees.

And there is a power and peacefulness in being in the moment, being grateful for each breath, and living each day like it's your last.

I have a friend who is living with a debilitating chronic disease. She told me that for several months she kept telling her young, athletic doctor that she feared that she was going to die. Shortly thereafter, on a ride without a helmet, her doctor died from a head injury when he fell off his top-of–the-line 24-speed bike. My friend has not spoken of death since then. Instead, she is grateful to be alive.

Another friend whom I met in a clinic was recently diagnosed with throat cancer. Such a diagnosis in and of itself is overwhelming enough, but in this case add to it the fact that he is a well-known singer and guitarist whose soul and essence are driven by music. Yet it is he who inspires me, not—though I try my humble best—the other way around. His enormously helpful, philosophical perspective hangs from my office door in the form of a handwritten note. It says, "Doc, all of us are living in the belly of the leviathan, and we have two choices: either we give up and perish, or we have hope and live!"

My choice is to have hope and live. It is scary as hell, and there are many nights that I wake up in a cold sweat after being visited by the ghosts of past sickly livers. But the fact is I do wake up. I am alive and that's a good thing. Sure, I have a vulnerable liver and sure, I have an eating disorder, but things could be worse. One day I know that I am going to die, and it could be from a bad liver. But not today. I'm not going to die today. Today I choose life. I will live today like it's the last day of summer. I will squeeze the life out of today like it was the last ripe orange on the planet. I also know that if you are anything like me—that is, a natural non-survivor—you, too, need a little help from your friends to get by. Together, we both have a tremendous resource in the work of Dr Sandra Cabot, as well as in the support and example of our family and friends, who will help us to find the courage that we need to accept our situation and to do whatever we have to do, no matter how hard and how frightening it may seem, to find health, and thus to find wellbeing.

CHAPTER THREE

The 10 P's

Almost everyone has at least one shining moment to look back on and view as the high point of his or her life. Sometimes the moment is dramatic, such as hitting the winning home run in the seventh game of the World Series, or heroic, such as the day of release from a POW camp, or particularly gratifying, such as the day on which one is recognized for one's accomplishments with an Olympic gold medal, Nobel prize, Oscar, or some other less prestigious award that is nevertheless treasured by the recipient. Conversely, there are people on this Earth whom circumstances have so unfairly humbled that their high point is the day on which a roof is finally put over their heads or real food is put into their distended bellies. For most of us, though, the high points are more pedestrian and ordinary, such as the day we give birth, graduate from school, get married, and the like. Unfortunately, these high points are not usually appreciated until well after the fact, during our not so high points in life when we tend to reflect on what really matters; moreover, the high points often come with regret associated with the fact that we could not hold onto that moment just a bit longer or appreciate it more thoroughly.

Paradoxically, my high point occurred on a high point. It was 2001, roughly two years after I found out about my fatty liver and about one and one half years after I found Dr Sandra's little green paperback book crumpled and nearly hidden between two encyclopedic hepatitis C narratives at a Barnes and Noble store in Paramus, New Jersey. On the fateful day that I found her book, I was fat, 40, and caught in the vise-like grip of a binge eating addictive behavior pattern. Miraculously, that little green book set into motion a series of events that culminated about 1,000 feet below the summit of Mount McKinley, the highest point on the North American continent, where I experienced the high point of my life to date.

My exuberance at reaching high camp on Denali (Mckinley's Native American moniker) was unlike anything I had ever experienced. After all, prior to 1999 I had spent my entire life sitting in any easy chair, playing spectator to the game of life. Never mind 19,000 feet, I don't think I had ever been over 1,900 feet—and then only by way of a car. In fact, the thought of mountaineering my way 19,000 feet above sea level, under my own power, carrying an 80 pound backpack, hauling a 100 pound sled, through treacherous crevasse fields and up glassy, exposed, steep glacial ice, in temperatures—and especially wind chill—far below 0° had not long before been as attainable in my mind as building my own arugula ship and becoming the first human to walk on Mars.

Only now do I appreciate the true implications of this accomplishment; and, as unbelievable as this may sound, the accomplishment itself had little to do with the mountain, or with the climbing. More importantly, none of my lingering regrets have anything to do with not reaching the summit. Rather, what I am able to see now, or rather appreciate now, with crystalline clarity, is the hidden value of a journey that extended over oceans and across expanses of God's most spectacular landscapes, involving some of the best and some of the worst people I have ever met.

For the culmination of this book, I would like to reconstruct this epic journey, which was ten years in the making. To do so, I have paired ten of my favorite adventures, all of which were made possible because of Sandra and the liver cleansing lifestyle, with my ten favorite life lessons, which I call "The 10 P's." The 10 P's are my homage to and version of the 12-step programs that have faithfully and consistently served addicts of all persuasions for decades. It is by means of the lessons of the 10 P's that I was able to turn my life and liver around; and if they can work for me, I assure you, they can work for you, too!

Neatly, the first five lessons deal with the theoretical world of addiction from a descriptive and recognition standpoint, whereas the last five are purely practical tools, tricks, thinking patterns and techniques to serve our day-to-day needs. For the sake of flow, these lessons and adventures are not always listed chronologically. For the sake of brevity, I have only included the portions of the adventures and lessons that I feel pertain to the spirit of this book. For the sake of collegiality and to avoid causing them embarrassment, I have either left out or changed the names of some of the less honorable players in my story. Finally, for the sake of truthfulness and authenticity, I have done my best not to exaggerate or exploit any of the situations to make myself look more competent or courageous. As a matter of fact, if you've been paying attention so far, I tend more toward self-deprecation than self-aggrandizement. I do this consciously so that you, my reader, never receive the false impression that I am acting as a guru, or that I have "it" all figured out.

If anything, I am a flesh and blood fractured mess of a man who, thanks to the efforts and experience of professionals, has the ability to share these stories to inspire my struggling brothers and sisters. In essence, I am the anti-guru, the person who stumbles when he walks, falls when he runs, and stutters when he speaks. Unlike the kitchy and postmodern "life is good" stickman who can be found on multicolored pastel tee shirts across the globe running or hiking or fly fishing with his trademarked "cat ate the canary grin," I tend to be more realistic.

Yes indeed, life can be good. As a matter of fact, sometimes it can be great. But it can also be ordinary, or scary, or challenging, or sometimes just plain bad—and, on occasion, downright tragic. So if I had to put my philosophy on a tee shirt, I would have my stickman doing all the same cool things with the same cool smile, but instead of "life is good" my slogan would read "life is sloppy."

Recently, new age superstar James Ray, author of one of my favorite self-help books, Practical Spirituality, hosted a sweat lodge at which several people tragically lost their lives. More locally, my childhood parish priest was spotted stocking produce at the local supermarket because of an indiscretion with a pretty churchgoer. Around the same time, my mother's favorite evangelical preacher lost everything because of fraud and embezzlement. Should examples like these convince us that every person in a position of spiritual or self-help leadership is full of shit? Absolutely not! Does this mean that if one of these leaders falls down, makes a mistake, or, better put, falls prey to "the sloppy life," everything that he or she has ever said or done should be ignored? Absolutely not!

I have read "The Secret" a dozen times or more, and I will continue to read it until the principles that I find valuable within it are absorbed. The same goes for the Bible, the tao, the Bagavat Gita, the Koran and about 1,000 other holy and sacred books. I also love Oprah, Eckhardt Tolle, James Ray and Wayne Dyer, and others who have dedicated their lives to making our lives better. And you already know how I feel about Dr Sandra...

But self-help gurus are not judge and jury for the rest of us. They are not gods to be worshipped. They are fellow humans, no better or worse than anyone else. And I'm sure that they would be the first to agree.

In the end, it is up to all of us to integrate their writings and philosophies with our own personal circumstances and life experiences.

It is up to us to seek out those who speak to our hearts and come up with our own synergetic personal philosophies and road maps.

That's what I have done here, on these pages—and, more importantly, in my life. I have taken a pinch of Sandra's commitment to curing the nefarious disease of fatty liver and a dash of my therapist's commitment to helping me to unravel the circumstances of my life that fueled my pathological behavior, and finally seasoned it with my life coach's insistence that I grow up and take personal responsibility for my life, and establish myself in an environment that will make me successful. What it all adds up to is this: Because we all stumble when we walk, and fall when we run, and stutter when we talk, the secret is to keep our balance, get right back up, and keep right on going.

Let's begin my sloppy adventure on the Appalachian Trail.

1. Perception and the Appalachian Trail

James Matthews is a cat. I say that he is a cat because I believe that he has at least nine lives. As a child, he was hit by a car and put in a coma. As an adult, he fell off a cliff and broke nearly every bone in his body. Again, he was put in a coma. Lastly, about seven years ago, shoulder pain prompted an x-ray that showed a large cancerous mass originating from his diaphragm. He had the tumor removed successfully at Memorial Sloan-Kettering Cancer Center, but he lost a portion of his lung.

You might think James would be a dire man, or an angry man, or have a huge chip on his shoulder. But that's only if you don't know James.

In fact, James is my hero. He is one of the most charming, loyal, and well-loved people on this Earth. It is therefore no surprise that James was the first person I called to help me out of my fatty liver funk.

Jim and I met in high school, freshman year, when each of us had to endure senior hazing with broken legs—he from an unsuccessful wrestling match with the above mentioned car and I from an unsuccessful gridiron encounter with a huge linebacker. We got to know each other fairly well in high school, but we quickly lost touch after that. I did remember, though, that Jimmy was a hiker. Not just an ordinary hiker, but also an Eagle Scout, and a passionate outdoorsman.

With my background growing up on a barstool or in a fast food drive-through lane, my primary intention was simply to get my fat ass into the woods. Who better to take me there than Jimmy Matthews? Unfortunately, what I did not realize was that two comas and extensive anesthesia had taken away the parts of Jimmy's brain that dealt with organization, logistics, and practicality—three fairly important skills when it comes to surviving in the wild!

I know that I should've recognized it when we met at the camping store to stock up on supplies for our first overnight trip: "Jimmy, don't you think ten pounds of cashews is way too much for overnighter?" And I know I should've recognized it when he forgot to bring a map: "No worries, Tom, the trail is well marked." But Jimmy was the so-called expert, so that's where I put my trust. Sounds reasonable, right? Wrong!

I was obese, out of shape, and weighed down by a pack that could have gotten me not only through the night but probably well into the following month. Each step up unfamiliar rocky inclines caused pain and suffering of a variety that I had never experienced. To make matters worse, we had no idea where we were, and it started to rain—which in and of itself is no big deal, unless you forget the tent fly, which of course we did...

I remember sitting in the tent shivering with cold, soaking wet, and hungry (of course, all of our food had spoiled in the dampness—even the ten pounds of cashews, which probably still lie where I threw them: at the bottom of Sunshine Lake!). Yet despite my uncomfortable surroundings, I found myself joyful: joyful that my journey toward health and adventure had begun, and even more joyful at the incredible opportunity and life lesson that presented itself—the lesson of realistic perception.

For the first time in my life, sitting in that obscenity of a tent, I finally was able to see things not just from my convenient "center of the universe" vantage point, but from a more fair and balanced perspective.

Suddenly, I wasn't as thin as I had thought, smart as I had thought, handsome as I had thought, healthy as I had thought, or as special as I had thought. I was just an ordinary overweight guy with a fatty liver who made himself out to be extraordinary in order to reconcile a bad self-image brought on by an unsafe upbringing. Talk about the emperor realizing how underdressed he was! I was downright naked and exposed, but for some reason, I didn't care. I was liberated to finally see the real me, without the protective wall of denial or the shield of rationalization.

I had been living in a world of ordinary perception for 40 years, a world in which we view ourselves, our environment, our circumstances, our philosophies, and even those around us in a very restricted and two-dimensional way. It was this two-dimensional thinking that inspired the blind trust that I had given to Jimmy to organize the camping trip. The truth was that I had no business setting off on such a trip without a modicum of physical ability, a map, food packed in waterproof containers, and a proper protective tent cover, not to mention limiting myself to a distance that I could realistically achieve without risking harm to life or limb.

The importance of this new found perception spilled over into other aspects of my life, especially as it related to how I viewed my addiction, my physical condition, and my role as master of a now self-directed rather than externally directed life journey and destiny. The blind trust that I had relinquished to Jimmy was the same blind trust that I had given to the physicians who were supposedly caring for my fatty liver. It was time to take matters into my own hands.

Why should any of us take a supporting role in any aspect of our lives? Should it not be our responsibility to advocate for ourselves and our job to protect our interests? After all, if not us, who?

After this epiphany, I became stronger and stronger with every hike I took—as well as leaner and leaner, and smarter and smarter. Never since have I let false perception put me in harm's way. Never since have I given anyone unilateral control over a hike, over my health, or over anything for that matter. Once one masters the power of perception a whole new world opens up, a world in which one becomes the master of one's circumstance and the authority over one's interactions. It is here that one's power begins.

Thankfully, Jimmy and I survived the day, and the night, and the next day. And luckily we did return to the good old Appalachian Trail, slowly making our way up the craggy Appalachian spine of the east coast one weekend at a time. So far, we have tramped from Maryland to Vermont. Will we ever conquer the entire 2,000-plus mile expanse? Probably not, but who knows? Crazier things have happened!

2. Priorities and Mount Hood

Did you ever see a movie or read a magazine article or a book that changed your life? Obviously, Sandra's little green liver book was life changing for me, but so was an article that I found in Outdoor magazine about 10 years ago. It was written by a guy a lot like me. Although he was a stockbroker and I was a doctor, we were both entering middle age and hovering between average to poor health. More interestingly, we both wanted to use travel and outdoor activities as our transformational mechanism.

It seems that this gentleman grew up in suburban Portland, literally in the shadow of Mt. Hood, and that climbing that beautiful peak had always been his dream. However, he was more inclined toward academics than sports, as was I, and after a high-powered college education he wound up working on the floor of the New York Stock Exchange. Suddenly, and for reasons that seemed identical to mine, he decided to change his life, and climbing Mount Hood was his goal. So he hit the Stairmaster around the same time that I was hitting the Appalachian Trail, and apparently we both came to the same conclusion: although slow, uncoordinated, unathletic, incompetent and highly comical when engaged in basketball, running, weightlifting, swimming or rowing, we both had a proclivity for slow, methodical, uphill movement that was a perfect fit for hiking and mountaineering.

By the time I read his article I had already become—albeit at an extremely slow pace—a fairly competent hiker, camper, and orienteer. But there was something that stirred in me when it came to the mountains. For one thing, the East Coast does not have real mountains—and when I say "real", I mean in the sense of the grandeur evoked by the scale and dramatic configuration of the Rockies, the Cascades or the Alaskan Range. Secondly, there has always been something extremely beautiful to me about snow and rocks and glaciers and jagged peaks. There was no question about it: I had to become a mountaineer.

I chose the same guide as the author, a gentle giant by the name of Mark. Mark was a true caricature of what I thought a mountain guide should be. He was tall, handsome, rugged, muscular and jocular. He looked like a linebacker, only happier. After introductions and the purchase of a whole new overpriced wardrobe of specialty gear, including spaceman boots with spiked crampons that theoretically would allow me to stick to the slippery steep slopes of the icy mountain, we walked slowly up to base camp, which was neatly tucked at the terminal end of the glacier that was to be our highway to the summit.

The weird thing about it was that I had hiked steep slopes before, but I was extremely short of breath and had a terrible headache. I almost felt like I was back with Jimmy on my first hike, even though I was in much better shape and was accompanied by an uberguide rather than by an uberflake. Little did I know at the time that I was paying the price for the panoramic views—in other words, I was suffering from the effects of high altitude. I thought that I was going to die, but Mark reassured me, set up the tent and the stove, and gave me some Advil, hot tea, and soup, and soon I didn't quite feel like my head was Keith Moon's bass drum.

On the second day, I learned the skill of self arrest. No, self arrest has nothing to do with sending yourself to jail; rather, it is a technique for using your ice ax to keep yourself from flying off the mountain if you happen to be unfortunate enough to slip and fall despite your crampons. In fact, I also learned how to tie knots, how to belay, how to walk with crampons, how to climb out of a crevasse, how to hold my ice ax, how to manage a rope, and how to crap in a bucket. I'm not proud of that last one, but boy is it necessary!

Most importantly I learned about silence and solitude. What many people, my former self included, do not know about mountaineering is that it's about 20 percent hiking, 20 percent food and shelter set up, 20 percent bullshitting, and 40% dead time. Thus, the real secret to enjoying mountaineering has nothing to do with the climbing per se, but rather with how you utilize your dead time.

At first, my dead time was filled with slaying my demons of fear. If you haven't figured it out already, if I were screen testing in Hollywood, I would not be competing for Errol Flynn-type roles, but rather for the sort of parts that Dom DeLouise used to play so humorously. Yup, everything frightens me, and being alone on a mountain, 10,000 feet above sea level, even with Jeremiah Johnson, did little at first to make me feel relaxed. Soon, however, with Mark's help, I actually began to enjoy myself. I started playing mind games, one of which was to try to quiet myself enough to allow entrance into a faux meditative trance. Once there, I tried to evaluate my life in an objective and non-judgmental way.

What I found was astonishing. I learned the crucial lesson of priorities, which made my lesson regarding realistic perception that much more meaningful.

For example, a person may discover his or her true three-dimensional footprint, and yet still not know how to use that information to improve his or her life. In my case, I finally discovered just how important and primordial an imperative it is to control my eating. I needed to give the devil—in this case my binge eating addiction—his proper due.

For 40 years I had been swinging the proverbial yo-yo between dieting and binging, with weight fluctuations as steep as 100 pounds. I had filled my liver to the brim with fat and was facing my father's ghost with reasonable expectations of an early death. Yet for reasons ranging from denial to fear of change, controlling consumption was still not a priority in my life. Sandra—who gave me my program, which gave me Jimmy and the Appalachian Trail, and the Outdoor magazine article, which gave me the sport of mountaineering, which brought me to Mount Hood—also gave me, via this chain of connections, the gift of priorities.

I have never met a mountain guide who was not fastidious to the point of being compulsive about safety. Each new adventure spawns a new guide whose idiosyncrasies and rituals vary. Yet even though the guides change the essence remains the same. They all keep their eye on safety. Safety is their overwhelming priority because without it, clients would die. They may die. So why wasn't I as definitive about my eating as they were about safety? Were the life and death stakes really any different?

The idea of elevating my "tripod" program of exercise, diet and learning, to my overwhelming first priority, was the true catalyst to the amazing adventure that my life was to become. I will not tell you that it was not difficult, and I will not tell you that it did not raise many eyebrows, and I will not tell you that it did not cause great consternation among my loved ones, but believe me when I tell you that if I had not prioritized my health and my program above everything else, I would already be dead.

How ironic it is that I spent so many years thinking how deplorable a disciplined life with food constraints would be, when actually a life of setting priorities and using restraint is infinitely more rewarding. Climbing Mount Hood forever changed my thinking—so much so that, as a reminder of that trip, I keep a framed summit photo on my desk. In it I am holding up my ice ax victoriously, trying to replicate the famous Everest pose of Tenzeng Norgay. Most of those who see the photo assume that my smile stems from the boisterous pride of personal accomplishment; in reality, it is the outward sign of insight and inner contentment.

3. Perseverance and Mount Rainier

I was built to climb mountains. I may be slow, and I may be a spaz, but I can climb all day.

One foot in front of the other—repeat one million times. After returning home from Portland, in short order I bagged many of the nearby Catskill and Adirondack high peaks. Yet after tasting melted snow on a glacier, I was eager to put my crampons back on. Mount Shasta and Mount Hood were great warm-ups, but I really wanted to go high, really high, and Mount Rainier is the highest point in the 48 contiguous states. It is a beautiful mountain, as they all are, but there is something extraordinarily special about the diversity of the wild flowers and brush of the lower mountain, the cute shenanigans of the wily marmots and the extraordinary breadth of the upper mountain, which has been said by many seasoned climbers to be reminiscent of the Himalayas.

As a matter of fact, many giants of postmodern mountaineering got their start on Mount Rainier, which stands a proud sentinel to the historically green, crunchy, and outdoorsy city of Seattle, Washington. I was eager to follow in their sacred boot prints, but instead of climbing alone, this time I invited a few friends. As most of you know, finding the right mix of personalities for an excursion of any kind is a treacherous and tricky proposition, even when friends are involved—or, perhaps I should say, especially when friends are involved! And, for some reason, my friends, the guide, and I did not mix well. There seemed to be some sort of cliquey division that brewed along lines of interest and ability. Add to that a severe bacterial infection known as cellulitis that had developed on my leg from a wasp sting, and soon the holy karma from Mount Hood had abandoned me.

So maybe it was the group, maybe it was my constant antibiotic induced state of nausea—or my fear demons—or maybe it was our guide, who turned out to be the complete opposite of Mark. He was short instead of tall, wiry instead of muscular and sarcastic instead of jocular. He also judged me on my pace, which made for a very bad interpersonal foundation. Summit day began at 3 a.m. with a bowl of oatmeal, which I quickly regurgitated because of nerves and nausea. The guide rushed us up a rocky traverse called Disappointment Cleaver (a perfect name, by the way) in order to stay clear of falling debris. But the pace and the altitude almost knocked me out of the game entirely. Again, I can go all day, but at the pace of a tortoise, not a hare.

At that point, I don't think any of us, including me, thought I stood any chance of reaching the summit. Finally, after an exhausting effort, we found ourselves at the crest of the rocks, literally at the Rubicon of the climb, when I experienced a burst of inspiration.

Maybe it was the rising sun in the eastern sky diffracting beautiful pastel light patterns from the lower clouds, or maybe it was the sugar rush from my p b and j sandwich, or maybe the bell rang just in time to prevent my knockout, or perhaps God sent down my guardian angel. Whatever it was, I learned the lesson of perseverance. Perseverance is defined as the determined continuation of an action or belief, usually over a long period, and especially despite difficulties or setbacks. Climbing Mount Rainier was a lesson in perseverance. A lesson in hanging tough and keeping up the fight despite whatever shit gets slung at you—whether it be an unpleasant guide, illness, fatigue, or all of the above.

And, as I usually do, I got to thinking. The hardest part of a climb or a change in diet or lifestyle is the beginning—before the sun rises, when the task at hand seems so enormous and undoable that one questions one's resolve.

For an addict, one must also take into consideration the physiological symptoms of withdrawal, and believe me when I tell you that detoxing from cheeseburgers hurts as much as detoxing from heroin!

Add to that the unbelievable despair that a morbidly obese individual endures knowing that it will take weeks or months of sacrifice before any visible results will begin to show. How many times do we throw in the towel and just say stuff it, and open the floodgates to hell. It is here, in this quagmire of hopelessness, that the food addict needs to persevere. It is here that one must draw that line in the sand, suck it up, use any tools, tricks and techniques—such as the last 5 P's—that can get one through to sunrise, to the point at which one actually believes that what one is doing is actually going to work, actually going to get one up that mountain, or flush that toxic fat out of one's liver, or—for those who wear them—get one into that little black velvet dress.

So, I bet you want to know if I made it to the top? Come on, be honest, you really do! Well, after that brief rest on top of the Cleaver, I strapped on my crampons and did what I do best: I climbed. I put one foot in front of the other and slowly made my way up that damn hill. At the false summit, which is right below the true summit, I began to sob, not cry, but actually sob like a baby. Of course, the horseshit guide thought I was in trouble again and tried to hold me back from continuing—go figure, right? But I would have no more of his nay saying. I didn't have the strength to explain to him that I had just done the hardest thing that I had ever done up until that point in my life, including medical school and parenthood. He most likely would not have understood anyway. I just passed right through him and his negativity like he was a vapor and went on to enjoy the view from the top of that splendid hill.

In the end, this achievement had nothing to do with

physicality: it was all mental. I was able to take a little green book, stay on a program of healthy food and exercise, train like an Olympian, and attain a peak unreachable without great preparation and effort, despite setbacks and obstacles, both real and imaginary. Afterwards, I decided to take the high road with both the guide and my friends. After all, it was not their job to understand me and my baggage. And it was not my job to teach them to. So we all celebrated our success in the good old American tradition of a toast and a meal—they with beer, wings, and steak, and I with seltzer and salmon. I could not have been happier. I had persevered!

4. Patience and the Seven Summits

In the 1980s, a wealthy entrepreneur by the name of Dick Bass climbed the highest peak on each continent. And although on the surface it seemed like a harmless happy game being played by some rich guy who had nothing better to do with his time and money, it actually changed the entire face of amateur climbing. However, the question of whether he changed it in a good way or a bad way is fodder for a debate that still rages to this day. For one thing, Bass opened up a niche for guided climbs up several very dangerous mountains. The short list includes some real notables. Mount Everest, the highest mountain in world, is extremely deadly; Mount McKinley, with her notorious weather, also has a deadly reputation; and Vinson Masif, located in Antarctica (how the heck does one get to Antarctica anyway?), is also not to be trifled with—and neither are Aconcagua, Kilimanjaro, and Elbrus for that matter, though, with all due respect to the folks down under, Mount Kosciuszko, Australia's high peak, actually isn't much of a stretch!

Let's face it, though, even if you are just climbing up a typical ski slope in the Caucasus Mountains, altitude and storms can make for a very bad day! Add to that the fact that climbing résumés and ability are trumped by cash, and you have the makings of a real tragedy—something that is well known to readers of Jon Krakauer's account of an Everest trip gone bad, in his book Into Thin Air. In any case, despite not having as deep pockets or as deep lungs as Dick Bass, I still wanted to give it a try—at least with the peaks that I felt were attainable.

The two that I tried were Mount McKinley in Alaska and Mount Elbrus in Russia. I failed on both.

But I did not fail because I was not strong enough, competent enough, or prepared enough. I failed because I lacked the patience and equanimity that were necessary to ultimately top out.

And please note that I use the word "fail" only in the most literal sense as it relates to reaching the summit. Actually, both trips turned out to be great successes in terms of life lessons, adventure, and experience. Remember, in the beginning of this chapter I told you that my life's high point occurred on Mount McKinley—despite not summitting.

So how can a failure still be a success? Sounds like an oxymoron, right? And how can a lesson as harsh as lacking patience actually be a good thing? Well, let us begin with the concept of patience as it relates to mountaineering, and then extend the lesson for those of us living life with a fatty liver or an addiction or both. Patience is a virtue. Who hasn't heard that cliché? But to have patience, and I mean true patience, is not only virtuous but also difficult as hell. And, on the surface, I seemed to have mastered even that bitch of a taskmaster.

Hell, to prepare to climb McKinley, I spent a year of my life slogging up local 1,300 foot Bear Mountain, sometimes three or four times over 16 straight hours of strenuous labor, to try to approximate the long climbing days that lay ahead.

I also did long multi peak climbs in the Catskills and Adirondacks, weight trained and stuck strictly to my diet.

My weight went all the way back to high school numbers and my liver functions went back to normal. I was literally a transformed man. And when I say transformed, I mean I should have been on Oprah. My friends and family really thought that I had been abducted by aliens: "Who are you and what have you done with Tom?" they would say. Yet there was still something missing. Remember, I mentioned my tripod—diet, exercise and learning. Unless all three legs are deployed, the apparatus will fall right over. For both McKinley and Elbrus, I had the exercise and diet down, but my head was off ever so slightly.

Yes, I had done the work. But it was in an artificial environment. When I landed on the lunar landscape of the McKinley glaciers, it was like nothing that I could ever have been able to even remotely reproduce. When push came to shove, and the weather went south, I let the influence of guilt from being away from my children and the impatience and personal agenda of yet another egotistical and self-righteous guide sway my resolve.

Bad weather on a big mountain is common and expected. It stands to reason, then, that delays of hours or even days hunkered down in a crowded and smelly tent are part of the price of admission. But it was here, in these delays, in my multicolored windswept polyester prison cell, that my mind went bad.

It was here, only 1,000 feet below the summit, at high camp, that I decided to raise the white flag.

Sitting here now, typing furiously on my computer, I lack a real answer as to why I decided to give up so close to the top. Maybe I thought that some day I would come back and finish the job. But the expression "I'll be back" hit its high points with McArthur and Schwartzenegger; it has yet to apply to me.

Maybe I thought that I was in over my head, had pushed myself to the brink, and didn't want to further tempt fate.

Maybe my guide's ambivalence and mind games were starting to gnaw at my confidence. Or maybe I just didn't believe that if I were patient and kept my cool, I would actually finish the job. Bingo; jackpot—we have a winner!!!

Having faith in what one is doing and believing that what one is doing will work is the core of the sixth P, Piety, which we will come to shortly. But patience and piety are close relatives. Ultimately, patience means the ability to figure out a way to stay perfectly focused on what one is doing, whether it's keeping one's mind still while waiting out a huge weather front at 18,000 feet for a week or more, saying "no" to bad food choices, or keeping to one's workout schedule despite not having broken through that oh-so-frustrating weight plateau.

Sometimes I wonder whether I would have summitted if I had not hit the bad weather in Alaska, or if I had not had to posthole-hike through waist deep snow in Russia (my private Idaho on that climb). But if I did, then I would never have had the opportunity to begin my work on patience. And if I hadn't been exposed to that lesson, my tripod would not be worth squat. I don't know about you, but life is hard enough as it is. I want as strong a tripod as I can get to help me through life's challenges and troubles. Having patience is a definite prerequisite to achieve this goal!

5. Paradox and Paris

Ok, enough about mountains. Let's talk romance. And if it's romance you are after, what better city to start with than the city of lights? In addition to mountaineering, hiking, running, skiing, and biking, my new Sandra Cabot liver cleansing lifestyle endowed me with enough vim and vigor to include cultural exploration along with my already hectic schedule. In a series of frenetic trips with my family, I zipped through French Polynesia, Europe, the Caribbean, as well as most of the high points of our American national park system, all while directing a busy cancer center in New York's Hudson Valley. I became known as the Tasmanian

Devil due to all the energy I put into everything that I did. I made people tired just by watching me.

In all my travels, I must say that I have a special place in my heart for Paris. Besides falling in love there, it is a city whose energy matches my own. With all its art, architecture, history, and intellectual tradition, it's no wonder that we have been back three times for long walks along the romantic boulevards, hot chocolate and roasted chestnuts in the Tuileries, and of course the bohemian splendor of the Left Bank. Unfortunately, it is also the city in which I learned the brutal lesson of paradox.

One day, while returning by train from an especially memorable exploration of the catacombs and an excursion to Versailles, I noticed that my pants were somewhat tight and uncomfortable. This perplexed me only because, in my mind, I had been perfectly on point with my tripod. My eating had been stable and binge free, I had been going to the hotel gym every day as well as walking the city like crazy, and my head was straight. I jumped on a scale as soon as I got back to the hotel, and low and behold, I had gained seven pounds. Now, usually I deserve my weight gains—I can normally even point to the meal or, even scarier, to the first bite of the culprit responsible for a multi-day bender. But in this case there was no smoking gun—not even a smoking burrito.

This experience freaked me out somewhat at the time, but as a result I stumbled upon the ultimate sad paradoxical truth regarding "foodies" like myself. Even when we are under control, our proclivity is toward weight gain. This is true partly because we often lack a good portion barometer and partly because we unwittingly tend to choose dangerous high carbohydrate options, and do not fill up on raw foods like salads, nuts, seeds and fruits and pure protein – instead we go for the addictive carbohydrates! Paris of course is full of tempting carby foods like croissants, pastries and high carb sauces. Even if foodies can somehow keep their portion amounts reasonable and appropriate, their wrong food choices quickly put their insulin levels up and voila – the liver must store fat.

Therefore, unless we can stay on track with our portions and palate and eat plenty of pure protein and raw foods we will slowly and covertly gain weight.

Luckily, this is not as bad an insight as you may think. For starters, knowledge is power, and this knowledge in particular is nuclear. Secondly, awareness of this fact can inspire us to maintain constant vigilance. Now, I know what you're thinking. There is absolutely no way that anyone can ever be constantly vigilant and mistake free. I agree, and, as I've said, I am the biggest cheater (P number 10) in the world. But I cheat without fooling myself – in other words without rationalizations or denial. I know all too well that for me to maintain equilibrium, I must do the work. The tripod needs to be equilateral and balanced.

Quite frankly, the cost of not knowing the truth is simply too high. After all, it's no secret why millions of people have fatty livers: we like to eat, and it's junk we like to eat the most. Sweets, fried foods, fast foods, refined foods—no matter what the quantity, and no matter if you have a food addiction or not, these are the basic building blocks of liver disease. Therefore, we need to be honest and truthful with ourselves at all times when it comes to what we are eating and how much.

We also need to realize that the epidemic of fatty liver is no longer confined to food junkies like me. You would be shocked to see how much fat a thin person's liver with a small appetite can hold if he or she lives on a typical western diet. So, I beg you to look deeply within yourself and make peace with the law of paradox.

6. Piety and the Adirondaks

Over the years, many people have been fascinated by my stories of adventure, especially people who knew me before my transformation. However, they seem less interested in the particulars of any individual trip than in hearing about my "near misses." For those of you who haven't figured it out, a near miss, at least in my case, has nothing to do with horseshoes or target practice. Rather, it has to do with the times when I came close to death. For instance, two hours after I pranced around the summit of Mount Hood, a medical student (of all things) fell from the summit to her death. Another time, two Brits following our rope train fell into a crevasse on McKinley, but luckily they were able to get themselves out.

Things like this happen all the time in mountaineering, I'm afraid, and they actually make for interesting "dead time" chat (no pun intended). In fact, listening to guides' conversation is one of the most bizarre things that I know. With one's eyes closed, they sound like South Florida retirees "one upping" each other with stories of how many friends they have lost in the last few decades. Then, one sees or remembers that they are in their 20's or 30's, not in their 80's, and one realizes that their friends died from shark attacks surfing in the Baja, not peacefully in bed or from choking on ill-fitting dentures. This realization makes the whole experience surreal.

That said, my closest near miss sometimes disappoints people because it had nothing to do with being extorted by machine gun carrying Russian soldiers at the Chechnynian border (which did happen), nor with almost having our small putt putt glacier plane kiss a mountain in bad weather (which also happened), nor with the time I fell off Grand Teton and swung like George of the Jungle into a rock face (yes, that happened too). Really, the only time that I think I was in actual peril—let me rephrase that: the only time that I really should have died occurred not on a 20,000-foot mountain in the Alaskan wild, but on a 4,000-foot hill in New York's Adirondack State Park.

As I mentioned, the Catskill and Adirondack Mountains

had become my playground and training zone. Combining natural beauty and rustic charm, I personally believe that they provide as stunning a backdrop as any other place I've been to. Yet hidden within their beauty lie dangers as severe as those of almost any place on earth. This is easy to forget, perhaps because the mountains are not gigantic, but make no mistake, the Adirondacks are deadly enough to merit the publication of a yearly morbidity and mortality report describing the grizzly outcomes of the dumb mistakes made by overconfident hikers like me...

Lest I digress further, here's the story: About four of us, headed into the woods on a beautiful, cloudless summer day. Our goal was to bag about three or four high peaks within an eight-mile loop. We figured that it would take us no longer than ten hours, taking into account my snail's pace. We even had a late dinner reservation at the lodge. Talk about overconfidence!

About four hours into the hike it started to rain and we laughed. About six hours into the hike it really started to come down in earnest, and we laughed harder. But by hour ten, after literally sliding down the summit of Slide Mountain like a water ride at an amusement park, we knew that we were in trouble.

We had become trapped within a flash flood in the middle of nowhere. No one even knew where we were, so there would be no help coming from the outside. And there was no chance that we could count on any other hikers, because I'm sure that any responsible hiker would have actually checked the weather report and cancelled his or her hike. We never even thought of checking the weather before a hike. After all, we were invincible. After all, several of us had hiked and climbed all over the world. We couldn't die in the measly Adirondacks, could we?

As we huddled to conserve heat, we enumerated our problems, which were plentiful. For starters, all of the cute little brooks and streams that we had easily rock-hopped over in the morning had engorged and become impassible. Secondly, hypothermia loomed large as we were wet and underdressed with the sun setting and the temperature stating to plummet. Lastly, due to the washout of the trail, we had to bushwhack through unfamiliar landscape in a best guess attempt to find our way out of the woods. Luckily, we found a tree that had fallen across one of the now deadly streams. If by some chance we could shimmy across the tree to the other side, we would have a fighting chance of getting home alive. If not, we would have to find a way to survive the night, of which there was no guarantee at this point. It goes without saying that we had no rope or gear of any kind that could have proven helpful...

As I was the least athletic, I went last. My three friends made it across, but it didn't look easy. I saw the fear of God on their faces. In fact, this was on my account because, as they tell me now, they really didn't think that I would be able to cross without falling in. After all, the tree was wet and slippery, and if I did fall into the water, it might as well have been filled with hungry crocodiles for all the chance I would have had of getting out again. Talk about pressure. Holy shit, I couldn't believe what was happening!

Slowly and gingerly I made my way across the tree. My heart was pounding so hard that I thought it was going to explode. Everyone was silent, so the only audible sound was the raging of the water inches below me. About halfway across I started to list to one side. I had to act instantly or I was going to fall, so I quickly disengaged my beautiful $200 Denali pack, and watched in horror as the water instantly swallowed it up, never to be seen again, car keys and wallet included. I regained my balance and resumed my crawl. Finally—it must have taken me 45 minutes to cross less than a ten foot expanse—I found myself being dragged off the tree and into the arms of my friends, who by that point were all crying and heaving up their energy bars.

Looking back on that night, which I have done over and

over and over again, there are several lessons that I learned—most of them so self-evident that I will not even bother to reiterate them here. Besides the obvious sins of neglect and hubris, I had never actually realized just how holy and pious an endeavor being in nature was. More importantly, I never understood how much humility and respect nature ought to command.

Yes. I had grown up as a city boy who never stepped into the woods until age 40. And yes, I had never received any formal Boy Scout or NOLWS training. But I had paid beaucoup bucks and spent a ton of time with world-class guides to take me to otherwise unreachable places, thus by now I should have known better.

When I started my quest to slay my food demons and fix my liver, nature was the first place that I went following Sandra's program. Basically, I spent all of my free time for several years exploring Mother Earth's amazing nooks and crannies. Yet despite all the experience I was gaining, I had never approached these activities with the proper respect, humility, or piety. Any addict will tell you that the first step to recovery is the recognition that one's demon is bigger than oneself and that one requires assistance from a higher power or creator in order to achieve one's goal. I had skipped that step. I had atheistically taken my lifestyle to Mother Earth, thinking that I was on equal ground with Her and capable of withstanding Her fury. Luckily, I enjoyed many years of dumb luck before that fateful day in the New York woodlands. Luckily, too, I survived the harrowing experience and escaped with what may be the most important lesson that I had ever learned. I learned that I needed to extend my piety and deference beyond my eating disorder to cover all aspects of my life, including recognizing the holiness and worthiness of my fellow men and women as well as that of all God's other creatures.

The practice of piety, together with the last 4 P's, is a practical rather than a merely theoretical consideration.

It is an active and integrative process that is original and individual to each of us. In general, though, it behooves us as addicts and/or sufferers from bad liver health to engage the help of a higher power. We need to recognize our limitations and to ask for help in whatever way suits us best—whether it be through prayer, meditation, chanting, singing, or reading. To me, the easiest way to engage or prime the engine of piety is by being grateful: there is no better way to get the attention of the universal creator than by engaging in the active expression of gratitude.

Often, when our lives are less than perfect, we find ourselves complaining. But what is it exactly that we are complaining about? Often those of us who complain the most are relatively prosperous, healthy, and gifted. Why, then, do we complain? I cannot stress how important it is to regularly complete one's gratitude exercises—though what these exercises consist of and when they work best for you will be yours to discover. For instance, I do my gratitude exercise when I wake up in the morning. The first thing I'm grateful for is just that: waking up. I then think about all of the blessings that I've been given. Lastly, I take stock of those around me and make comparisons. I'm sure that you, too, can easily find examples of people who suffer greatly. This knowledge and insight brings us closer to our creator and helps us to become closer to those around us.

Needless to say, my friends and I survived the night and walked safely out of the woods. But we did so in silence and respect rather than with laughter and bravado. We all knew that we had cheated death, and we needed time and space to place this knowledge appropriately within our souls.

After several more hours of walking, the lights of a small cabin appeared in the 1 a.m. haze of what had become a new day. I will never forget the look of shock and amazement that the ranger wore on his face when he opened the cabin door. And I certainly will never forget his words: "When I saw your headlights I thought you guys were either the luckiest sons of bitches I ever saw—or the dumbest!"

The only thing I could retort in my exhausted and dazed condition was: "Guilty on both counts".

7. Prevention, Preparedness, and the Ironman

"Swim 2.4 miles! Bike 112 miles! Run 26.4 miles! Brag for the rest of your life!" is the registered trademark of the Ironman competition. Begun in 1978 to settle a bet as to whether swimmers or runners were the ultimate endurance athletes (biking was added in 1982), U.S. Navy Specialist John Haller completed the first race in just over 11 hours. Since that first race, which attracted about one dozen Hawaiian locals and no fanfare, press coverage, sponsors, or spectators, the Ironman has become the yardstick against which endurance athletes measure their abilities. Naturally, too, it became the event on which my crosshairs were focused.

After all, I had gone from a half dead couch potato to a jet setting mountaineer, biker, runner, hiker and world explorer; why not become an Ironman? Since implementing my liver-cleansing tripod, my weight had dropped from 300 to 183 pounds, my body fat was down from 40% to 17%, and my liver enzymes were all back to normal. I figured that if anyone had the horses to complete this race, it would be me, right? Wrong! Unfortunately, what I had not encountered up until year seven was failure. And when I say failure, I don't mean not getting to the summit of a mountain type of failure—I mean big time reversion to my old ways.

One of the many problems with addiction is the constant threat of falling off the wagon. Even addicts who give the proper respect and have the proper resolve, addicts who work their programs every day, are at risk. It's just the nature of an addiction. That's why one hears stories of alcoholics passing the same neighborhood bar everyday for 26 years and not going in, and then one day, for no apparent reason, they walk into the bar and order a drink.

I have a hiking buddy who goes by the name El Camino Joe. He is an alcoholic. He hasn't had a drink in 17 years and most likely will never have another drink in his life, but he will emphatically tell you that he remains an alcoholic. One day I asked him to explain this concept to me. After all, I had beaten my food addiction, hadn't I? I was six years food "sober," in remarkable shape, and looked at least ten years younger than my actual age. I had healthy kids and loyal friends. Why would I throw all that away for cheeseburgers and pizza? I mean what kind of ass slaps God across the face by returning such a gift? Again, guilty as charged. But I needed to go through my fall from grace just like everyone else, ugly and painful as it might be.

Today, the analogy that Joe used sizzles in my memory center like a quality steak on a Weber grill. But at the time it was just another cute story. It seems that while escorting his wife to her office Christmas party one year, Joe was asked to fill in for the no-show bartender. His wife, who never knew him when he was drinking and clearly didn't realize the potential conflict, unthinkingly volunteered his services. Luckily, Joe declined. The way he saw it was that the risk that he would resume drinking far outweighed the embarrassment that his wife would feel for hosting a lame, bartenderless party. She was naturally furious and refused to speak with him the rest of the night. However, in the morning cooler heads prevailed and she was open to his explanation, which he kindly passed on to me:

Most people who do not understand addiction continually try to subject me to their interpretation of what is safe and unsafe behavior. I have even had people implore me to join them in a toast—'Come on, you haven't had a drink in 17 years'—or for a beer while watching the Superbowl—'Come on, one beer isn't gonna kill you'—or even something as seemingly innocent as a sip of wine at Communion—'are you kidding me, it's the blood of Christ, for Christ's sake!' But what my wife and all the others don't understand is that I don't want just one sip of champagne or one drink at a bar, what I want is to be swimming in a huge pool filled with vodka. And if I take just one sip, that's exactly where I will try to go: to the pool filled with vodka!

At the time, Joe's story was moving and scary, but not relevant to me yet. I was basically a narcissistic ex-foodie who was above all of that addict stuff. And I was going to be an Ironman!

So I signed up for the Lake Placid Ironman, hired a coach, and of course bought more expensive gear. Interestingly, the value of my bikes surpassed the value of my car! I was getting pretty serious. But the truth of the matter was that doing an Ironman competition was too much even for me. The training absolutely kicked my ass, and I got very frustrated with all the little wear and tear injuries that were not severe enough to stop my training but painful enough to be discouraging. Mind you, I had done many really crazy and extreme endurance activities, but Ironman is something way outside even my box. In the end, I did manage to swim 2.4 miles, bike 112 miles, and run 26.4 miles—just not on the same day!

The silver lining was being able to compete in several sprint and Olympic distance triathalons (the same idea but over shorter distances), which I found to be a hoot. But my disappointment about not successfully getting to the starting line at Lake Placid was a hard pill to swallow, and as a result I began to swallow other things.

Slowly, I began to introduce some of my old trigger foods, such as fast food and sweets. Even though I was still working out, my weight climbed slowly, demonstrating the paradox explained earlier: that a foodie's equilibrium is set toward weight gain, which will take over whenever complacency sneaks in. The irony was that while I was participating in the sport of triathalon, there was a lesson right in front of me that, had I taken notice of it, I would have been able to right my ship immediately, instead of spending my entire post-

Dr Sandra year seven, scrambling to get back to baseline. That lesson is the P of prevention and preparedness. In my mind, there is no better preparation process—athletic or otherwise—than preparing for an Ironman competition. And there is no sport that is better suited to setting up careful systems to prevent catastrophe.

By definition, the Ironman is an event that pushes one not only to the cusp of mental toughness, but to the brink of physical capability as well. There have been elite triathelites who have gotten to within yards of the finish line only to pass out from exhaustion, dehydration, and electrolyte imbalances. And yes, very fit people have died attempting the Ironman. In addition, since the event is multisport, it involves dangerous transition zones. Within these transition zones the athletes need to switch outfits, feed, and hydrate, all within a ludicrously short span of time. Failure to dry off completely puts them at risk for chaffing and skin ulcers, the pain of which can escalate unbearably over a 17-hour day. Failure to drink or eat enough, too, puts participants at risk for cramping at best and for multi-organ failure at worst.

If you watch these elite athletes train as I have, you will notice not only an unsurpassed level of intensity, but an almost insane level of attention to the details of their preparation and prevention measures. And the reason they are so fastidious to their routines is simply that they know that they have to be both physically prepared and mentally able to deploy preventive strategies, lest they risk dropping out of the race or, worse yet, becoming injured.

El Camino Joe knew that he needed to be prepared for circumstances like his wife's Christmas party, and his calculated refusal of what seemed a simple request prevented a circumstance that could have ended his 17 years of sobriety—or even his life. Yet the majority of us addicts, myself included, fail to appreciate the necessity of such a disciplined and often inconvenient lifestyle. And for the food addict, again, there is the extra layer of complexity brought on by having to dip into the kettle of kryptonite multiple times a day!

For myself, after countless failures, I think I finally know what I need to do to prepare for and prevent a binge. I have even kept a ten-year food and exercise diary, and the patterns that it reveals are eerily distinct. First off, I have categorized the environments in which my binges arise, and have found that over 80% occur after either taking a first bite of a trigger food, eating within a crowded environment such as a party—especially when it is an event that I am hosting—or on days when I fail to work out. Yet this begs the question as to how far a food addict should go to prevent a binge. For example, if I know that I stand a significantly increased chance of starting a binge if I attend a social engagement, why don't I just stop attending them? Such a tactic appears simple enough when one thinks of elective crowds like when a bunch of work pals get together at TGIF's for a beer and some wings. But what about gatherings that are mandatory for one's career or family? Would you have the strength and heart to tell your daughter that you won't be attending her high school graduation party or, worse yet, her wedding? In such cases, do we just throw down the gauntlet and ditch? Or do we show up and risk a binge?

More difficult are the other 20% of binge days, which I attribute to the "blahs." The blahs are what one feels on days when everything just seems a little bit off. Problems at work, not feeling well, fight with the spouse, busted boiler, or bent fender—the instigating point is irrelevant. The question is just how far can the blahs take you before you just say stuff it and give in to the cravings?

Lastly, and most importantly, is the alarming statistic that my binges are seldom single day affairs—meaning that, in my experience, only 10% of the time can one stop the binge after one day. If you are lucky, maybe you can stop at two days. Personally, my eating diary shows that the average number of days it takes for me to reverse the spin of a binge is 3.4. That's a lot of food and a lot of calories, especially when we all know how long it takes to lose 20 pounds and how quickly it can be gained back—not to mention the distinct possibility that the binge will never be reversed!

So what is one supposed to do? I've raised more questions than I have answered, perhaps because like most of us I haven't completely mastered my feelings about food. This, however, is what I suggest:

1. Try to eliminate the first bite of trigger food whenever possible.
2. If you fall prey to the first bite of trigger food —pause (P number 10).
3. Eliminate all elective social events.
4. Attend mandatory social events only after a hefty work out.
5. Never allow yourself to fall into no-win situations.

Let's look at that last point more closely. Remember, one always has a choice—sometimes it just takes planning and preparation. For example, if your workplace does not have a cafeteria that serves healthy, non-trigger foods, buy a small dorm-type refrigerator and prepare your own meals and snacks. In fact, it's usually best to take the same approach to mandatory career and family functions. I long ago lost count of all the office parties, bar mitzvahs, graduations, weddings, and communions that I have brown bagged to avoid the trigger foods that cluster ominously around these events! Also, one may have to attend a family wedding, but one sure doesn't have to stay for the cocktail hour, which is like being a kid locked in a toy store overnight who must refrain from playing with any of the toys. Finally, be creative with your preventive behavior: spoil yourself by spending an extra buck or two on a quality meal, and please don't worry about looking stupid—your creative healthy choices can actually be a great topic for conversation!

As for the Ironman competition, I doubt now that I will ever achieve that milestone, and I might as well scratch it off my bucket list. The half-Ironman, however, is a totally different story!

8. Palatability and Biking through Europe

Growing up in a city, I didn't have much use for a bike. We got around fine by walking. And where we couldn't walk, we took the bus.

One Christmas morning, however, my mother surprised me with a bright green Raleigh chopper 5-speed. It was absolutely gorgeous. She must have had to work three weeks of overtime to afford something so fancy.

For those who are not certain what a "chopper" looks like, it had a small tire in the front and a big boss tire in the rear. The movie Easy Rider had just come out in the cinema and every time I straddled my new hog I fantasized that I was Peter Fonda on his Captain America bike.

The only problem was that the bike was cursed. Honest to goodness, nothing ever good came from that bike. First, I almost killed myself going down a steep hill. What I didn't know at the time was that in order to slow a bike down quickly, one has to use the back brake since the front brake will more often than not simply throw the rider over the handlebars. Yes, I did fly through the air with the greatest of ease—until the laws of gravity reapplied and scraped off most of the skin off my chest and off my chinny chin chin. I wear facial hair to this day to hide the scar.

Shortly after my stitches healed, the bike was stolen. I guess I wasn't the only kid who thought the bike was bitchin'. I wonder if the thief is still alive...

Later, when I went to college, I met a few fellas who were planning to do a cross-country bike trip. The plan was to leave New York the day after spring semester, ride the 3,500 or so miles to San Francisco, and fly home in time to start the fall semester. They had a ball, the pictures were awesome,

THE LIVER THROUGH A MICROSCOPE

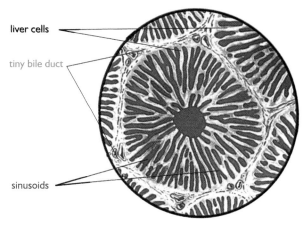

liver cells

tiny bile duct

sinusoids

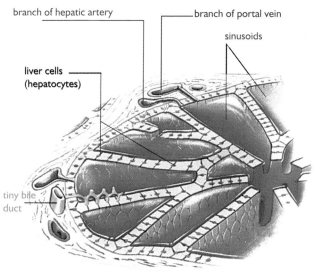

branch of hepatic artery

branch of portal vein

sinusoids

liver cells
(hepatocytes)

tiny bile
duct

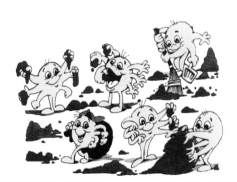

Dr Cabot's cartoon of
KUPFFER CELLS

*These are specialized
liver cells that live in the
liver filter. They ingest
and destroy rubbish
that would otherwise
contaminate your blood.*

Dr. Sandra Cabot

Left: Dr Sandra Cabot and Naturopath Christine Ki on the road in Arizona doing a health seminar tour.

Below: Dr Cabot is a pilot and donates her time and plane to Angel Flight Charity.

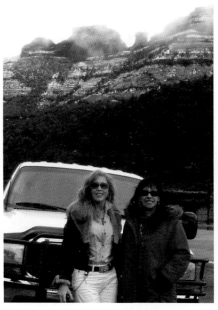

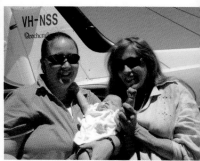

Dr. Thomas Eanelli

Below: Before improving his liver function and lifestyle.

Right: Looking and feeling strong and healthy in the great outdoors.

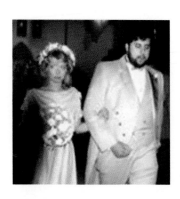

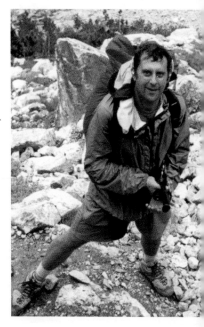

and yes, I was jealous. But being the conscientious pre-med student that I was, it was never the right time to do stuff like that—or so I thought. Besides, I used my fat meat suit as an excuse to build an impenetrable wall around me.

When I finally got thin on Sandra's program, I wanted to find an activity that I could share with my wife. Hiking, mountaineering, and endurance trials are not her thing. She loves travel and culture and beauty, but she likes to experience them in a relaxed and controlled manner. Being that I had been born again in a new body and with newfound stamina, however, I was not content to stroll the cobblestone streets of walled medieval cities until each one melted into the next. I needed to find a compromise—thank God for Backroads!

Backroads is a company that puts together hiking, strolling, and biking trips through the nooks and crannies of the world. In addition to the breathtaking scenery, they supply a sag wagon that allows people to bike as little (my wife) or as much (me) as their hearts desire. They also fill the trips with interesting and like-minded people, so the conversation is always stimulating—and the food is "to die for".

So began our exploration of Europe. The first year found us biking across Portugal from west to east. Through the cork farms and olive groves, through the small town squares with overlooking castles, vineyards, and ranches, we biked and ate our way all the way to Spain. Year two took us through the verdant Tuscan countryside, where the hills are steep and the wine and pasta pure. Most recently, we hiked and trekked our way through the Swiss Alps and biked the Interlaken countryside, energized by an awesome diet of fondue and raclette.

If you haven't picked up on it, there is a "work hard, play hard" theme to my story. But balance is also crucial, especially as it relates to food addictions and fatty livers. So let's pause for a moment for a brief quiz that I call "True or false and name the appropriate P":

1. A thin person can have a fatty liver.

2. All of the foods that I just listed are probably considered "trigger foods" by most binge eaters.

3. No matter how much exercise you do, if you don't watch what you eat, you become what you eat.

And here are the answers:

1. True (P number 1: perception)

2. True (P number 7: prevention and preparedness)

3. True (P number 9: portions—see below).

Ok, touché, I appear to be contradicting myself when it comes to the safe approach to trigger foods, but that's because we've only just started on the eighth P: palatability.

Palatability is the rule that acknowledges that no matter how successful a program may be, whether it is Sandra's liver cleansing diet or some other nutritionally sound regime, if everything that you eat tastes like cardboard, then the sustainability of your program will be limited by your tolerance for bland, awful food—and no one can tolerate bland, awful food forever!

With this in mind, consider the Backroads model. One's entire day revolves around an activity that is calibrated to suit one's level of ability. And, as an added bonus, the views are heavenly, in sharp contrast to the four walls of a gym. Lastly, one is sustained by a diet of European ambrosia, with each regional specialty lovingly prepared and slow-cooked by professional chefs.

Active lifestyle and slow cooking are the secrets to the success of this model, and also the reason why Europeans are on average considerably thinner than Americans and Australians.

In all three trips—Portugal, Italy, and Switzerland—we never ate any fast food or junk. All of the food that we ate was either picked from the farm that same day or purchased fresh at the local market. Inconvenient, yes; but very healthy!

In addition, all foods were prepared using natural and freshly pressed extra virgin olive oil, with no saturated trans fats, margarines, or synthetic corn syrup. The portions were respectable but not overdone. And there was a balance between proteins and carbs, with sweets mostly taken in the form of fresh fruit.

We were there for the exercise to be sure, but our exercise was somewhat contrived. I mean, we specifically traveled thousands of miles just to be in an area that had great biking or hiking, and although I resumed my regular active lifestyle when we returned to the States, I was in the minority. After all, I know a lot of people, and yet I am the only person I know who bikes to work. In Europe, almost everybody walks or bikes, whether one is a five-year-old student or a 90-year-old barber. In Amsterdam, they have so many bikes that they need parking garages to house them: tens of thousands of bikes—it's a beautiful thing!

For the most part, too, Europeans do not belong to any chi-chi health clubs, they do not hire trainers, and they do not sign up for five-kilometer races. They are active by virtue of a slow and simple lifestyle that is mirrored in their cooking; it's a lifestyle in which they tend their own gardens, do their own chores, clean their own houses, and build their own sheds.

This is what I aspire to. I aspire to a slower life where the food is natural and delicious and one's activities are pure and strenuous. I wonder what percentage of authentic, old school, slow lifestyle Europeans have fatty livers. Probably very few!

9. Portions and the New Jersey Shore Marathon

When I was a teenager in the 1970s I got caught up in the jogging craze that took the United States by storm. I started with short distances, one or two miles around an outdoor high school track. I thought that I was the coolest thing on the planet as I fantasized about being Bill Rodgers winning the Boston Marathon or Steve Prefontaine winning Olympic gold. Let's face it running circles around a quarter-mile track is enough to turn anyone delusional!

I also started reading Runner's World. It was, and still is, a great magazine, filled with tips on everything from healing blisters to carbohydrate loading and from running fast to running long. But out of all the articles, my favorites were those that had anything to do with marathons—from historical accounts of Phidippides running the 26.4 miles from Marathon to Athens, after which (having recently run to Sparta and back) he expired from exhaustion, to the improbable victory of Frank Shorter in the 1972 Munich Olympic Games. Yet in those days there was a mystique that formed a huge elitist barrier to the race. Although the distance did keep it out of the reach of all but the heartiest athletes, it was more the philosophy of logging huge numbers of miles per week—often over 100—for months beforehand that caused shin splints and tendonitis galore, squashing more than a few hopes and dreams—as did the unspoken rule that if you ever had to stop running, even for a minute, to work out a cramp or take a sip of Gatorade, you were committing treason of the highest degree.

Happily, the leukemia and lymphoma society of America—whom I call the Purple People thanks to their bright colored jerseys—had an idea. They thought that they could make the race less formal by turning it into an inspiring fundraiser and by introducing the concept of the walk/run. Soon, a flood of articles touting manageable running schedules appeared everywhere, sporting titles like "Get Ready for Your First Marathon in Just 15 Weeks". The basic concept was simple: short runs on alternate days followed by one long weekend run, which steadily increased from week to week until one got to 20 miles, followed by a taper to avoid injury, with the percentage of the mileage covered by walking and by running varying from program to program.

To the chagrin of the running purists, the walk/run idea quickly caught on and, more importantly, brought the marathon down from the stratosphere to within the reach of the ordinary Jill or Joe. Soon, hundreds of teams representing every disease and cause imaginable, each with its own colorful uniform, flooded the races, with runners ranging in size and shape from petite banana to chubby pear, often with pictures of the children or adults for whose sake they were running pinned to their shirts. It mattered little that the customarily respectable time of four hours or so crept up to five, six, eight hours or more. Ordinary folks were crossing finish lines all over the world to the cheers of the throngs who applauded their determination and selflessness.

Some races, like the Philadelphia Marathon, maintained a strict time limit and took down their road markers as soon as the bell curve passed by, leaving the turtles to fend for themselves—something that actually happened to me. Other races, like the Rock and Roll Series, became "penguin friendly" thanks to the exhaustive efforts of John "The Penguin" Bingham, who became the patron saint of the slow and challenged. Soon after, marathons everywhere opened up to anyone who had a desire to complete their dream race giving me my shot at the run that I had fantasized about for 30 years. The venue would be the Jersey Shore Marathon because it was flat, friendly, and in my home state.

The next several months were crammed with a running program that I had researched on the Internet. Unfortunately, my hiking stamina and mountain endurance did not translate well to running, so I had to work hard to even get into run/walk shape. But with patience (P number 4) and perseverance (P number 3), I got ready just in the nick of time.

When the fateful day arrived, I found myself at the "early start" line for the slowbos—a feature that some of the races offered as a courtesy to the turtles so that they would not end up finishing alone in the dark with no support stations. What I hadn't expected, however, was to find myself in the middle of an Overeaters Anonymous meeting.

> *Everybody at the early start line was overweight except for me, which blew my mind because it had always been I who was the porkiest pig everywhere I went.*

For the first time, because of Sandra and the liver cleansing lifestyle, I was not only thin and fit, comparatively I was emaciated!

In fact, the folks around me looked like they were waiting for the Olive Garden to open up for Sunday brunch, not for the sound of a race gun. And they were eating voraciously before they even took a step: bagels, cream cheese, peanut butter, energy bars and goos of every variety were being thrown down their pie holes with expediency reminiscent of the yearly July 4th Nathan's hot dog eating contest. I knew at once that I had to talk to these former brethren and find out what the hell was going on. How could they reconcile the paradox (P number 5) of being fit enough to run a marathon but rotund enough to be mistaken for a beach ball? Apparently, however, there was no such conflict going on in their minds, as they did not even pick up on the point of my somewhat indelicate questions about the race and their fuel. The closest I got to an answer was the admission that, indeed, they tended to gain rather than lose weight during these runs, which is mind-boggling when one considers how many calories must be consumed to not only replace but overshoot the huge amounts of energy necessary to power their large frames for six or more hours of strenuous activity.

Expecting the proverbial light bulb to appear overhead like

a sign from God, I was seriously disappointed when all I got back was deer-in-the-headlights, lobotomized looks of confusion while jaws continued to shred food at a furious pace. And then I remembered the lesson of portions taught to me as an adolescent by my Uncle Butch. After church on Sundays, Uncle Butch would take us to a diner, which is a very dangerous place for a foodie owing to the scope of the menu. Perhaps it was the immaturity of my young but already food addicted mind, but I became conflicted over having to choose between pancakes, grilled Taylor ham and cheese, or an omelette. Sensing my struggle, Uncle Butch did me the "favor" of ordering all three. Now you don't need to be a dietician to know that there is a limit to how much a 12-year old can safely eat without becoming ill, even a binge eating, food addicted 12-year old. As I recall, on the first such occasion I consumed about one-third of the gluttenous feast before I excused myself to purge. In his booming voice, Uncle Butch told me in no uncertain terms that my eyes were bigger than my stomach and that I had better take notice. I can still feel the embarrassment of that moment to this day.

But, as I said, it was a great lesson. One of the reasons that fatty livers are so common is because of our gluttenous portions—portions so big that fatties even gain weight while running a marathon. The western diet has been criticized for decades for the size of its portions, yet its supremacy around the globe is growing at an alarming rate.

If you think about it, how much food does one really need in order to fill up? At restaurants, do we really need to eat the 20-rib slab plus the appetizer and dessert to be satisfied? When I was climbing Mount Elbrus in Russia, there were no fast food restaurants or big super-duper grocery stores. Our peasant cook put a brown bag lunch in our packs that consisted of one sandwich, one apple, a small chocolate bar and as much mountain water as we could carry. On summit day, we got an extra apple. There were no scientifically formulated energy drinks or space-age sports bars or goos. And, believe it or not, it was enough.

Now, when I go to a restaurant, I order a soup or salad and an appetizer for my main course. And, believe it or not, I—once the king of the Chinese buffet—leave perfectly satisfied. So, if you find yourself reading this book because your liver has mysteriously filled up with fat, try portion control ASAP!

By the way, I finished that first marathon in five hours. Since then, I have run the New York City Marathon twice, as well as eight other marathons from California to Vermont. One day I hope to have run one in every state. But thanks to Sandra and Uncle Butch, I never expect to gain weight during a marathon.

10. Pause and Grand Teton

Pause, the last of the 10 P's, is the most crucial and the most useful for turning oneself around during a slide. It doesn't matter if the slide is caught at the very first bite of a would-be binge or after years of neglect, when we finally listen to the painful cries coming from our swollen liver. Unfortunately, by analogy to the degrees of mastery that one attains while studying martial arts, the lesson of pause is the liver-cleansing equivalent of a seventh degree black belt, which eludes all but the most devoted and serious of students.

Believe me when I tell you that after a decade of living the program, I have journeyed from the cellar of human despair to the roof of human accomplishment and back again. But because I am "roped in" or better yet "on belay" from the 10 P's—particularly the P of pause—I may fall but I will not crater (yes, to crater means exactly what it sounds like: to fall off a mountain and make a crater in the ground where one lands). To be "on belay" means that while one person is climbing, the other is positioned to catch that person if he or she falls. But because no human can actually absorb the full force of a free fall, the gear and rope take advantage of the wonderful laws of pulley physics to diminish the otherwise unmanageable brute torque to a manageable brisk tug. Metaphorically, that's what Sandra and her liver program—and these 10 P's—represent: our belayers. Without the program's systems, recipes, menus, snacks, liver tonics, insights, and techniques I could never have made such a remarkable turnaround without cratering. And if you didn't need a belayer to catch your fall, you would have never bought this book! We all need a little help now and then. That is nothing to be ashamed of. As a matter of fact, needing help is part of what makes our human journey human.

When I climbed Grand Teton, I was at the top of my game. I was in year six of my program, at my all time low weight and pinnacle of health. But I was not a technical climber. Even my extreme mountaineering experiences had been garnered on relatively gear-free "walk ups"—trails that did not require rock skills. So I was very excited to add yet another dimension to my expanding set of outdoor abilities.

Jim Williams is a world-class guide whose list of first ascents, Himalayan climbs and high altitude rescues is the stuff of legends. And the three days that I spent at his "rock school"—learning how to master a rope like a cowboy, master gear like batman, and master a whole new vernacular of skills—were as demanding as military boot camp; but wow, how rewarding! One of the skills with which I had the most trouble was repelling. Repelling is the act of gingerly yet intrepidly climbing down a rope. Now I know that sounds much easier than climbing up a rope, but believe me when I tell you that the first time you allow yourself to give up all control and lean back over a cliff's edge with nothing between you and a 3,000-foot drop to your death but some knucklehead and a piece of fancy synthetic rope, it takes every bit of self-control not to start crying and soil yourself.

I steadied myself, leaned back and let go. Soon, I was G.I. Joeing my way down to safety, screaming with delight. I passed all of my requisite drills and was ready for another 3 a.m. summit-day wake up call.

We began our technical ascent well before sunrise on day four, this time with me holding down my oatmeal like a champ. Headlamps punctuating the blackness were all that one could see before sunrise, which was fine by me, an ostrich to the core. But when the sun did rise and we stated to climb, it became progressively easier to reconcile this uncomfortable exposure to such narrow ledges and deep drop offs. Halfway up, I was showing some real skill on fairly steep faces with knobby little holds. Jim must have been proud, as I definitely had not proven myself a rockstud on the previous three days. Finally, on the last pitch, my nerves caught up to me and I became frozen. Jim made his way over to me and taught me the lesson of pause.

Rock climbing is a wonderful and highly addictive sport that combines grace, strength, intelligence, nifty technical gear, and the opportunity to become one with the rock. Most importantly, I believe that it is the necessity of complete interdependence and trust with one's climbing partner that softens the rock-hard edge of this extreme sport. In any case, because there is a limit to the amount of rope that one can carry, and due to varying route heights, most climbs get divided into pitches. For example, a short climb up a relatively easy route in New York State's Shawangunk Ridge—widely known as The Gunks—may require only three pitches, whereas a complex route up Yosemite's famous El Capitan may take dozens. Each pitch requires a leader to set up the protective gear and a belayer to prevent catastrophe. This gear acts in tandem with one's partner's expertise to arrest a fall. Since both the mechanical and the human element are necessary, however, one's partner literally holds one's life in his or her hands, and vise versa.

Between each difficult pitch in a climb comes a brief pause.

It is here, in this pause, that one regains one's physical and mental strength, both of which are necessary to climb a tall rock. In a life spent caged by an addiction, there are many moments—and I mean many moments each day, not just each year—when one's courage and resolve will be tested, much as mine were tested by that last pitch on Grand Teton. But if we just pause to catch our breath and balance, we can avoid a binge.

Jim told me to close my eyes and visualize what I needed to do—to actually see the line of moves and series of holds that would allow me to heave my tired body over the top and onto the summit of that awesome piece of rock. And that's exactly what I did: I visualized myself taking the actions that I needed to take; then I executed them identically to my visualization.

That, moreover, is precisely what I'm telling you to do next time your cage gets opened. I want you to take a moment to pause. I want you to take a moment to breathe. And I want you to take a moment to visualize how awesome you will feel and how great you will look if you just stop the binge in its tracks, before it has the chance to demoralize you while in sight of your goal!

CONCLUSION

If your latest binge has already started, do not worry. You are on belay. Enjoy whatever piece of fried or sugary treat you have in your hand, then pause, and regroup. The secret is to stop the process at one bite, one meal, or one day.

After the pause, it will be necessary to return to your powerbase. My powerbase happens to be a work out. Sometimes I will literally stop a binge in its tracks after one bite or one meal by doing an agonizing hike up Bear Mountain or 20 miles on my mountain bike. Personally, I can think of no more empowering an activity than activity to get one's head straightened out!

In your case, maybe your powerbase is meditation, or calling a friend or an addiction mentor, or watching a dumb funny movie to divert yourself from temptation. But whatever your powerbase is, get to it as soon as possible.

On the other hand, if this is the first time that you are coming to terms with your addiction, or if you have only recently been informed about your fatty liver, again do not worry: you are also on belay. I know that this may sound incredibly artificial and contrived, but I believe that you are at the cusp of a life-changing and life-affirming journey on which you will look back with great pride and satisfaction. This will be your chance to climb that high peak of personal growth and to hit that high note of fulfilling your human potential.

That said I doubt very much that you are in the mood to consider the shock you may recently have received with anything other than fear and anger. I know—I've been there! And again, if you've bought, borrowed, begged, or stolen this book, you are looking for a place to start.

First, attack the obvious. Engage your mind. Begin reading as much about fatty liver and liver health as possible.

Use Dr Sandra Cabot's books, your personal physician, a liver specialist (hepatologist), the internet or the American Liver Foundation (www.liverfoundation.org) or any other sources that you will find helpful. Always remember that knowledge is power, and you need as much power as you can get to overcome what has most likely been a life of self neglect and wrong choices!

Thereafter, engage your heart. Look deep within yourself and ask the question: Why? Why do I have a fatty liver? Why do I have a liver disease of any type? Why do I have a food addiction? Why do I drink too much alcohol? What path led me to this book? You already know this author's story, so ask yourself: What is mine?

If you are part of the growing fraternity that has fallen prey to a high carbohydrate and processed westernized diet resulting in a fatty liver and yet you do not have an eating disorder or addictive behaviors, then Dr Sandra's tips will get your liver healthy in no time. But if you are like me, a food addict with a ton of baggage, you will need to dig deep—deeper than you have ever gone with introspection or even with personal counseling or psychotherapy.

If this is the case, then I recommend that you work your way up the ladder of the Ten P's. If you are reading this book, you already have a modicum of perception, but do you have the tenacity to make your program the overriding priority in your life? Do you possess the perseverence that will be necessary to endure the hard times when everything around you, including your entire belief system, is crumbling? Can you be patient enough to allow the program time to take root and show measurable results, and then find even more patience when you hit a snag or find yourself stranded on a plateau? Will you be able to accept the paradox that your program is a lifelong commitment, not a quick fad to get your blood chemistries leveled or to make you look good for a special occasion? Will you be devout and pious enough to view your work on this program as sacred and to be willing to express your gratitude regardless of whether you feel grateful at any given moment? Can you be vigilant enough to be prepared, no matter what the circumstances, to prevent a slide—to dip into the kettle of your kryptonite every day, three times a day, to enjoy wonderful and palatable food, but in reasonable and balanced portions?

If we are honest, the obvious answer is "not always," and that's OK because it is the truth. Our lack of consistency and the fallibility of our judgment have been proven time and time again throughout human existence. But if we can master the last P, the P of pause, maybe, just maybe, we can put a little space and a little time between our desires and our actions, we can keep as much mastery over our weaknesses as possible—and, at the end of the day, that should be enough. Let's stay clear of the pool of vodka—or, in my case, the cheeseburgers—at all costs. But, more importantly, let's not crucify ourselves if we slip into the hot tub of hot dogs every so often...

I also encourage you to generously supplement the 10 P's with whatever feels right in your gut, whether it be a 12-step program, a spiritual program, artistic expression, or getting close to nature. Give yourself some room to think, to feel, to purge. Tears are common—embrace them. Let your mind plan, but let your heart lead.

In my case, one of the "places" my heart led me to was the writing of this book. To be fair, however, I have been pretty comfortable asking you, the reader, to look deeply within your soul for truth, so I ought to do the same when it comes to what I have just written and why. Is it a self-help book, a new age novel, a diet book, a professional monograph, or just a longer version of the Sandra Cabot testimonial that I quoted in the Introduction?

For starters, it definitely is not a medical treatise, as I am not qualified as either a liver specialist or an addiction counselor. Moreover, despite having come down from the mountains to study writing at Columbia University and fancying myself as the next Ernest Hemingway or John Steinbeck, I know that this is not the great American novel, which nevertheless lies somewhere within the deepest recesses of my being.

Which leaves self-help book, new age novel, diet book, or testimonial? Now, I think, we are getting warmer. Yet, to be honest, I think that the book is either none of these things or all of them simultaneously. I therefore classify it as a "new age heal fatty liver-weight loss testimonial" and expect that you will be able to find a copy at your local bookstore ironically sandwiched (pun intended) between Fatty Liver for Dummies and The Zen Art of Binge Eating Control.

Now that we have settled the classification question we can ask: for whom did I actually write this book? I recently met with another writer to discuss a possible collaboration on a cancer survivorship workbook. He came to the meeting with his little notepad filled with appropriate and seemingly rudimentary questions about the project, such as the intended audience, possible interested publishers, and the EP—that is, the "earning potential" of the book. Yada yada yada. I started to laugh. He seemed a bit annoyed and insulted, so I made up some lame excuse about a cute thing that my 12-year-old daughter had done in school that day, which spontaneously ripped me up.

But the fact remained: I had just given six months of my life to this fatty liver/binge eating confessional, and I didn't have a friggin clue who would even be interested to read it. Was it intended for the person who had just been told that he or she has a fatty liver and is scared out of his or her shoes? Or did I write it for the closet binge eater, or the Twinkie junkie, or the closet drinker or to set myself up as the John the Baptist of fatty liver evangelists?

Maybe the answer is that I had to write this book for myself. After all, the God's-honest truth is that, at the age of 50, I still cringe when someone touches my belly or calls me "fatso." At the age of 50, I still cringe at the negative or "invisible" receptions that obese people receive. At the age of 50, I still cringe at the assumption of stupidity and weakness that an obese person must endure every time he or she meets someone new. At the age of 50, I still cringe at the disgust with which obese people are met by the public at large. And, at the age of 50, I most certainly still cringe at the discrimination that an obese person must endure in the workplace.

And if these feelings are still so raw and powerful in me, what will become of an increasingly large and younger generation of people who suffer from fatty liver? Just the name "fatty liver" is enough to give me pause for concern and fear of all the jokes, snide remarks, and callous comments that await my fellow sufferers. So I guess that my fame in life won't be as a great doctor, patient advocate, world explorer and adventurer, father, friend, or husband. By writing this treatise, by baring my soul and putting my neck on the chopping block, exposing my most sacred, intimate, and monumentally personal and embarrassing moments, I have unilaterally nominated myself as the poster child for fatty liver.

And so it goes. Here I stand, naked for all to see. The fat kid from Paterson, New Jersey, whose drunken father screwed him up so badly that he had to resort to food to quench his fears and drown his insecurities, ends up with a rotten liver from a gluttenous lifestyle. Serves him right. Or does it?

It is time for someone to stand up and fight back. It is time to stop having to explain to everyone that one is not a pig. It is time for people with food issues and resultant liver problems to disengage mortification and to get the help that they so richly deserve in order to live a free and healthy life.

I am here to say "No, you don't have to be ashamed of your disease. No, you are not grotesque and unlovable. No, you are not unworthy of help"

I am here to help you—and Dr Sandra and her team are here to help you. I know that you are going to have a hard time believing this, but I truly believe in my heart of hearts that this book is not a new age ponzi scam trying to take advantage of the vulnerable. We don't have a contract, we do not have an agent, and we do not have any immediate plans to jump on Oprah's couch!

We are here to stand up for you. We are here to demand mainstream medical attention for a ubiquitous and deadly disease and to give a credible voice to naturopathic and nutritional medicine. We also aim to foster holistic, practical and inspirational help for all the shamed and lambasted food addicts all over the world.

Incredibly, it's already working. Fifteen years ago Dr Sandra Cabot's work was ridiculed and judged unworthy by a closed and complacent traditional medical system, with relatively no money being invested in fatty liver and NASH research, and even more crucially into childhood obesity prevention programs. Just last week, however, I received the following email from the American Liver Foundation:

Education is the most powerful tool we have to prevent liver disease. In 2009, it has been estimated that up to 6% of school-age children are suffering from non-alcoholic fatty liver disease (NAFLD), a condition that can lead to diabetes, liver cancer and even liver failure. That's why we need your help.

The American Liver Foundation (ALF) has developed the Love Your Liver Youth Education Program specifically geared toward children aged 5-17 years. This program speaks to children in an age-appropriate way to educate them on liver wellness. In 2010, we need to reach as many children as possible with this life-saving program.

www.liverfoundation.org/chapters/yep

Can you imagine a world in which fatty liver will be as huge a public health concern as cancer, heart disease, and diabetes?

As someone with liver issues stemming from behaviors that started before I was ten years old, this email was the sweetest news I have ever received!

At the end of the day, fatty liver disease of all degrees can be eradicated if we educate and embrace those who suffer—whatever the reason: social and/or psychological—and remove the stigma of judgment and superiority that surrounds the disease.

I believe in this collective work and I have seen the effectiveness of Dr Sandra Cabot's theories and methods on regaining liver health. Because of her work and the care of other colleagues, I have been to the Promised Land and have been given a life that can only be described as magical. No, I am not perfect, and yes, I have strayed—but never far enough to keep me out of the woods or off the mountains.

And if I can do it, I know that you can too!

God bless you on your journey, and I hope to see you out there one day, walking the Earth, enjoying the journey, climbing mountains both literal and metaphorical, and adding new chapters to our story of passion, excitement, struggle and success.

Thomas Eanelli MD

www.confessionsofafatman.com

References

FATTY LIVER

Nonalcoholic fatty liver disease P. Angulo, Chapter 34 GI Epidemiology, Blackwell Publishing Ltd: UK Publication date: May 2007; ISBN: 9781405149495 http://www.blackwellgastroenterology.com/9781405149495.

Geoffrey C. Farrell, Nonalcoholic fatty liver disease: From steatosis to cirrhosis, Hepatology 2006;43:S99-S112

Younossi Z, et al. Nonalcoholic Fatty Liver Disease: An Agenda for Clinical Research. Hepatology 2002;35:746-52

Ratziu V, et al. Liver fibrosis in overweight patients. Gastro 2000;118:1117-23

Clouston A, et al. Nonalcoholic fatty liver disease:is all the fat bad? Int J Med 2004;34:187-91

Chitturi S, et al. NASH and insulin resistance: Hepatology 2002;35:373-79

Brunt EM, et al. Nonalcoholic steatohepatitis: A proposal for grading & staging the histological lesions Am J Gastroenterol 1999;94:2467-74

Taurine - Orthoplex Research Bulletin, "Taurine the Detoxifying Amino Acid", Nutrients in Profile, by Henry Osiecki, Bioconcepts Publishing, Brisbane, Australia.

Dandelion- Australian Journal of Medical Herbalism, Vol 3 (4), 1991.

MILK THISTLE

Lang I. et al., Australian Journal Medical Herbalism, Vol 4 (1), 1992.; "Effect of the natural bioflavonoid anti-oxidant silymarin on superoxide dismutase activity".

Muzes G. et al., Biotechnol Ther: 263-70, 1993.; "Effect of the bioflavonoid silymarin"

Carini R. et al., Biochem Pharmacol 43:2111-5, 1992,"Lipid preoxidation, protection by silybin"

Talalaj - Research paper, Silybum marianum, Sydney, NHAA, 1985.

Muriel P, Prevention by silymarin of membrane alterations in acute CCL4 liver damage. J Appl Toxicolgy 1990;10(4):275-9.

Saller R, et al. The use of silymarin in the treatment of liver diseases. Drugs 2001;61(14):2035-63.

Flora K, et al. Milk thistle (silybum marianum) for the therapy of liver disease. Amer J Gastroenterol 1998;93(2):139-43.

Pares A, et al. Effects of silymarin in alcoholic patients with cirrhosis of the liver: results of a controlled double blind, randomized & muticenter trail. J Hepatol 1998;28(4):615-21.

Wellington K, Jarvis B. Silymarin: A review of its clinical properties in the management of hepatic disorders. BioDrugs 2001;15(7):465-89.

Skottova N, et al. Silymarin as a potential hypocholesterolaemic drug. Physiol Res 1998;47(1):1-7.

Krecman V, et al. Silymarin inhibits the development of diet-induced hypercholesterolaemia in rats. Planta Med 1998;64(2):138-42.

Trinchet JC, et al. Treatment of alcoholic hepatitis with silymarin. A double-blind comparative study in 116 patients. Gastroenterol Clin Biol 1989;13(2):120-4.

Ferenci P, et al. Randomised controlled trial of silymarin treatment in patients with cirrhosis of the liver. J Hepatology 1989;9(1):105-13.

Wagner H. Antihepatoxic flavonoids. Progress in Clinical and Biology Research. 213:319-331,1986

Diseases of the Liver and Biliary System. Dr. Sheila Sherlock, Blackwell Press

Bland J.S. et al. Nutritional up-regulation of hepatic detoxification enzymes. The Journal of Applied Nutrition, 1992, 44; No. 3 & 4

Professor Robin Fraser et al, Lipoproteins and the Liver Sieve. Hepatology 21:863-874. 1995. http://www.chmeds.ac.nz/~ grogers/liver98.html

Cells of the hepatic sinusoid, Vol. 5.,Kupffer Cell Foundation, P.O Box 2215, 2301 CE Leiden. The Netherlands.

Ito T. Recent advances in the study on the fine structure of the hepatic sinusoidal wall. A review. Gumna Rep Med Sci 1973;6:119-163

Wisse E, et al. The liver sieve: considerations concerning the structure and function of endothelial fenestrae. Hepatology 1985;5:683-692

Lieber CS, et al. Role of dietary, adipose and endogenously synthesised fatty acids in the pathogenesis of the alcoholic fatty liver. J Clin Invest 1966:45:51-62

SELENIUM

Margaret Rayman et al, "Dietary Selenium: Time to act", The British Medical Journal, Vol. 314, 387-388, February 1997

Margaret P Rayman, Review: "The importance of selenium to human health". Lancet 2000; 356:233-241

Selenium and HIV, Arch Intern Med 2007;167:148-154 (Hurwitz BE, et al)

Rayman MP. The argument for increasing selenium intake. Proceedings of the Nutrition Society, 2002 May; 61(2):203-15

Linus Pauling Institute Micronutrient Research for Optimum Health Oregon State University

Dworkin BM. Selenium deficiency in HIV infection and AIDS. Chem Biol Iteract 1994;91:181-6

Combs GF Jr. Reduction of cancer mortality and incidence by selenium supplementation, Medizinische Klinic (Munich,Germany) 1997 Sep 15;92 Suppl 3:42-5

Clinical Insight, Selenium, Bioceuticals, Vol 55 August 1009

Selenium as a Chemopreventive Agent in Human Primary Hepatocellular Carcinoma, Yu S Y, Proceedings of STDA's Fifth International Symposium. 8-10 May, 1994 Brussels

JUICING REFERENCES

Fujioka, K. Research presented at Potential Health Benefits of Citrus Symposium. Philadelphia. 2004.

L. Tappy et al. Comparison of thermogenic effect of fructose & glucose in humans Am J Physiol Endocrinol Metab 1986:250: E718-E724.

Dulloo A, et al. Efficacy of a green tea extract rich in catechin polyphenols and caffeine in increasing 24-h energy expenditure and fat oxidation in humans. Amer J Clin Nutr 1999; 70:1040-45

Le QT and Elliott WJ: Hypotensive and hypocholesterolemic effects of celery oil may be due to BuPh. Clin Res 1991; 39:173A

FATTY LIVER IMAGING TESTS

Stanley RJ, Biello DR, Levitt RG, et al, Computed tomography of the liver. Radiology 1978;127:159-163.

Bashist B, et al, Computed tomo-graphic demonstration of rapid changes in fatty infiltration of the liver. Radiology 1982; 142:691- 692.

Quinn SF, Gosink BB. Charaterstic sonographic signs of hepatic fatty infiltration. Am J Roentgenol 1985;145:753-755.

Scatarige JC, Scott WW, Donivan PJ. Fatty infiltration of the liver: ultrasonographic and computed tomographic correlation. J Ultrasound Med 1984;3: 9-14.

Foster KJ, Dewbury KC, Griffith AH, Wright R. The accuracy of ultrasound in the detection of fatty infiltration of the liver. Br J Radiol 1980;53:440- 442.

Behan M, Kazam E. The echographic characteristics of fatty tissues and tumors. Radiology 1978; 129:143-151.

Taylor KJW, et al, Quantitative US attenuation in normal liver and in patients with diffuse liver disease: importance of fat. Radiology 1986;160:65-71.

Gosink BB, et al, Accuracy of ultrasonography in diagnosis of hepato-cellular disease. Am J Roentgenol 1979;133:19-23.

Caturelli E, Costarelli L, et al, Hypoechoic lesions in fatty liver. Gastroenterology 1991;100:1678 1682.

Scott WW, et al, Irregular fatty infiltration of the liver; diagnostic dilemmas. Am J Roentgenol 1980;135:67-71.

Schaffner F, Thaler H. Non alcoholic fatty liver disease. Prog Liver Dis 1986;8:283-298.

Yoshimitsu K, Kuroda Y, et al. Noninvasive Estimation of Hepatic Steatosis Using Plain CT vs. Chemical-Shift MR Imaging: Significance for Living Donors. J Magn Reson Imaging; 2008;28 (September): 678-684

Fatty Liver Clinical Study - www.liverdoctor.com/study

Index

RECIPE INDEX

Is your liver a ticking time bomb?

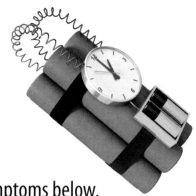

If you tick 5 or more of the symptoms below, you may be one of the many Americans who suffer from liver problems -

- [ ] Fatigue
- [ ] Body odor
- [ ] Bad breath
- [ ] Pot belly
- [ ] Unexplained weight gain
- [ ] Inability to lose weight
- [ ] Allergies
- [ ] Depression and/or moodiness
- [ ] Headaches, esp. associated with nausea
- [ ] Indigestion/intolerance of fatty foods
- [ ] Overheating of the body

- [ ] Excessive sweating
- [ ] Abdominal bloating and congestion
- [ ] Discomfort or pain over the liver
- [ ] Reflux and/or heartburn
- [ ] Hemorrhoids
- [ ] Fatty yellowish lumps in the skin
- [ ] Skin problems - psoriasis, eczema, hives or itchy skin
- [ ] Red itchy eyes
- [ ] Gallstones or gall bladder attacks
- [ ] High blood levels of cholesterol and/or triglycerides
- [ ] Multiple chemical sensitivities

Potential benefits of improving your liver

- Better fat metabolism for easier weight loss

- A reduction in levels of blood fats - cholesterol and triglyceride

- A reduction in blood pressure

- Better immune function

- A reduction in headaches including migraines

- Increased energy levels

- Clearer and less puffy eyes

- A reduction in allergies and chemical sensitivities

- Clearer skin with a reduction of brown liver spots and rashes

- A reduction in blood sugar levels

- Less moodiness and a clearer mind

- Improved digestion

- Less abdominal bloating

- Less constipation

More healthy recipe ideas can be found in Dr. Cabot's recent book titles

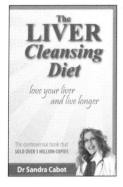

The Liver Cleansing Diet
Revised Edition

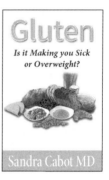

GLUTEN
Is it making you
Sick and
Overweight

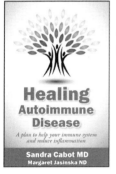

Healing
Autoimmune
Disease

I Can't lose Weight
...and I don't know why

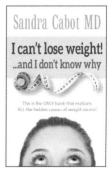

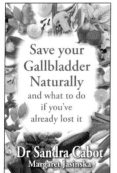

Save your
Gallbladder
Naturally
and what to do if
you'vealready lost it

Do you need a liver function test?

Ideally, everyone should have a liver function test done annually; these tests are even more important if:

- You take long term medications, especially several drugs at one time, or a lot of pain killers
- You have a family history of liver disease
- You drink more than 2 alcoholic drinks everyday
- You have high levels of iron in your blood
- You have had tattoos or body piercing
- You have had a blood transfusion before 1987
- You are diabetic
- You are very overweight
- You work with chemicals
- You have used recreational drugs/ shared needles